A System of
Scientific Medicine

A System of Scientific Medicine

Philanthropic Foundations in the Flexner Era

Howard S. Berliner

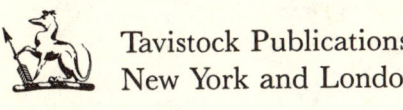
Tavistock Publications
New York and London

First published in 1985 by
Tavistock Publications
in association with Methuen, Inc.
29 West 35th Street, New York NY 10001
and Tavistock Publications Ltd
11 New Fetter Lane, London EC4P 4EE

© 1985 Howard S. Berliner

Printed in the United States of America

All rights reserved. No part of this book may be reprinted or
reproduced or utilized in any form or by any electronic,
mechanical or other means, now known or hereafter invented,
including photocopying and recording, or in any information
storage or retrieval system, without permission in writing
from the publishers.

Library of Congress Cataloging in Publication Data
Berliner, Howard S., 1949–
  A system of scientific medicine.

  Bibliography: p.
  1. Medical education—United States—Endowments—
History. 2. Medicine—Research—United States—
Endowments—History. 3. Endowments—United States—
History. 4. Medical education—United States—History.
5. Flexner, Abraham, 1866–1959. Medical education in
the United States and Canada. I. Title. [DNLM:
1. Flexner, Abraham, 1866–1959. Medical education in
the United States and Canada. 2. Foundations—
history—United States. 3. History of Medicine, 20th
Cent.—United States.   WZ 70 AA1 B49s]
R745.B45 1985   610'.7'1173   85-14724

ISBN 0-422-79520-8
ISBN 0-422-79530-5 (pbk.)

British Library Cataloguing in Publication Data
Berliner, Howard S.
  A system of scientific medicine : philanthropic
  foundations in the Flexner era.
  1. Medical education——United States——History
  I. Title
  610.7'1173   R745

ISBN 0-422-79520-8
ISBN 0-422-79530-5 Pbk

For my mother and father:
Marion Levine Berliner and Simon Berliner

Howard S. Berliner
April, 1985

Contents

Foreword	ix
Acknowledgements	xi
Introduction	1
1 From Philanthropy to Foundations	**7**
The changing political economy of the United States—1860–1900	10
The Gospel of Wealth	13
2 The Growth of Higher Education in the United States	**19**
3 Frederick T. Gates and the General Education Board	**26**
The General Education Board	28
4 Medicine in Chicago	**35**
The University of Chicago–Rush Medical College Affair	36
5 The Establishment of the Rockefeller Institute	**53**
6 Gates and Medicine	**76**
A brief digression on the germ theory of disease	79
7 The Reform of Medical Education	**92**
The Carnegie Foundation	97
The American Medical Association Committee on Medical Education	98

8	**Abraham Flexner and the Flexner Report**	101
	Flexner and the Carnegie Foundation	103
	The Flexner Report	111
9	**The Response to the Flexner Report**	118
10	**Foundations and Medical Education—1910–35**	128
	The growth and upgrading of the hospital	133
11	**The Full-time Plan**	139
	The struggle for the full-time plan at Johns Hopkins Medical School	146
	The 1911 Report	148
	Full-time after Osler's letter	154
12	**The Full-time Plan Expands to Other Schools**	162
	The American Medical Association and the full-time plan	164
	Medical systems in Europe	166
	Flexner, Gates, and scientific medical education	169

Notes on the Archival Sources   176
References   178
Index   185

Foreword

This is a fascinating book—a description that, to the best of my recollection, I have never before applied to a scholarly inquiry into health policy or any other realm of social policy. For academic inquiries do not generally enthrall readers, however much they may educate and enlighten. Dr. Howard Berliner's monograph does all three: it educates, enlightens and in so doing, is utterly fascinating.

The theme, "Philanthropic Foundations in the Flexner Era," hidden behind the title, *A System of Scientific Medicine*, scarcely suggests the intellectual excitement, institutional conflicts and important societal issues that are in store for the reader of Berliner's book which is based on a skillful reconstruction of primary source material. The author's use of diaries, letters, and other autobiographical data has helped to make this study a rare treat from academia.

All of the principal personae come to life — the Flexners, Abraham and Simon; the Rockefellers, both Senior and Junior; Gates; Osler; Harper; Welch and many more of the turn-of-the-century greats. Each of the principals was a big man—big in vision, strengths, determination to have his own way. The conflict among these giants creates the backdrop for the drama that Berliner traces in detail yet avoids overloading his text with minutiae.

But while big men and their struggles create the preconditions for exciting drama, it is the core issue over which they contend

A System of Scientific Medicine

that transforms the story and captures the reader. Rockefeller Senior was a devotee of homeopathic medicine. His principal philanthropic advisor, Frederick T. Gates, a former Baptist minister, perceived that the future depended on "scientific medicine" and, once convinced, marshalled supporters to his cause, including Abraham Flexner and John D. Rockefeller, Jr.

This is the battle of institutions—The Carnegie Foundation versus the Rockefeller philanthropies, and later a struggle to the death on the General Education Board between Gates and Abraham Flexner.

The issues are not trivial—the reform of American medical education and latterly, the appointment of full-time clinical chiefs at the nation's leading medical schools. And throughout, we find the philanthropoids determining through their granting and withholding of gifts the future path of United States medicine. The medical profession followed their lead.

Indicative of the high drama, let me call attention to but one episode: the great Osler leads the fight of the clinicians at Johns Hopkins against the reformers, Gates, Flexner *et al.*, and while he forces a delay he loses the battle and then the war. Those students of health policy who have any intellectual curiosity about how American medicine catapulted itself into a position of leadership after World War II with the support of the National Institutes of Health will want to broaden and deepen their understanding of the formative period on which the latter scenario was founded —when two men, Flexner and Gates, using the Rockefeller fortune, set the stage for this mid-century triumph.

Eli Ginzberg
Director
Conservation of Human Resources
Columbia University

Acknowledgements

This book draws very heavily on my Doctoral thesis at the School of Hygiene and Public Health at the Johns Hopkins University. All of the acknowledgements and thanks for help and inspiration for that tome still apply today. There are, however, additional people whom I would like to thank for their particular contributions to this book.

The University of Chicago Library, The Rockefeller Archive Center and the Oral History Research Office at Columbia University have all been generous in allowing me the use of the materials which form the basis of the research presented in this book.

Jack Salmon, Robb Burlage, Miriam Ostow and Eli Ginzberg were kind enough to read and comment on an earlier version of the book. To them I owe a debt that will take a long time to repay.

I would also like to thank Gill Davies of Tavistock for her encouragement throughout the process of writing and producing this book.

To my sons, Erik and Jeffrey Berliner, I owe the time I spent working on this book. Their patience, love and assistance helped to make this an easier project than it could have been. Peggy Clarke is owed the greatest debt of all. Her love and support were matched only by her editing zeal. I hope that the future will allow me to show her the love and respect I feel for her.

Introduction

In 1910, the Carnegie Foundation published Bulletin Number Four entitled *Medical Education in the United States and Canada*, which was written by Abraham Flexner. The Flexner Report, as it has come to be known, has been credited with transforming the American medical education system from one of the worst in the world to one of the best. Yet, three-quarters of a century after its publication, the exact process through which this change in medical education evolved remains shrouded in mystery. Moreover, there are indications that many of the worst practices that were highlighted by Flexner and presumably excised from the system forever, have returned to haunt contemporary medical education.

As late as the early 1890s, Americans who wanted to study the most advanced approaches to medicine were forced to go to Europe to do so. Bacteriology, physiology, micro-anatomy and a host of other scientific approaches to the study of human disease were simply not taught in medical schools in the United States. There was no medical research, with the exception of the occasional physician who established a laboratory in an office or home. Medical schools were predominantly proprietary, that is, they operated on a for-profit basis with the faculty essentially owning the school. The qualifications for acceptance into medical school were negligible, when there were standards at all. Physicians were not highly regarded and their incomes were, at best, on a par with mechanics. Disputes over the value of particular medical therapies

A System of Scientific Medicine

and approaches to disease existed throughout the country. The internecine sectarian warfare among allopaths, homeopaths and other practitioners that permeated the American health system did not foster public respect for the institution of medicine.

By the 1920s, and certainly by 1930, the situation had changed almost completely. Students who wished to pursue the latest developments in medical research could do so in the United States and in some cases foreign students came here to study. A host of privately endowed research institutes competed with well-equipped universities and medical schools for the best research talent the nation could produce or import. Medical schools required a full college education for entrance and medical schooling lasted an additional four years which did not include a hospital internship and possible residency. Physicians gained respect as scientific leaders in the community and their moral authority reached well beyond the strict confines of medical practice. Physician incomes began to rise in tandem with popular respect and both incomes and public opinion of the profession reached heights that would have been considered unimaginable only a generation before.

This rapid transformation of American medicine is without equal in any other field over so short a time. It is the Flexner Report which has been most frequently credited with acting as the catalyst for this change, if not creating the change by itself.

An observer of the American medical educational system in 1985 might see many of the same patterns that prompted the Carnegie Foundation into action seventy-five years earlier:

— A growing surplus of physicians raising fears of unnecessary care, skills erosion and charlatanism.
— Estimates that at least 7,500 physicians with bogus medical credentials practise in the United States.
— The recent establishment of off-shore medical schools, (primarily in the Caribbean), unaffiliated with universities or hospitals, which are proprietary in nature and have marginal admissions standards.
— Much debate over the nature of the medical school curriculum and the lack of scientific method in what is taught.

Introduction

— A growing sense that too many physicians are unacquainted with the latest scientific developments and discoveries, leading to inadequate and substandard patient care.
— The need to import third world physicians into the United States to work in under-served inner city and rural areas.
— The increasing incidence and prevalence of malpractice litigation resulting in part from physician performance being at levels lower than public expectations warrant.
— The increasing utilization of self-care and alternative care modalities implying a growing public dissatisfaction with physicians and with medical practices.

These concerns with the current state of American medical education emphasize the need to re-examine its development; to fully comprehend the process through which medical education initially changed and to understand the limitations of attempts to replicate that same process.

There are many facets to the Flexner Report that limit the ability to reproduce its effect in medical education or in other fields. These would include:

1 The recommendations of the Flexner Report were implemented by an external source (the Rockefeller General Education Board [GEB]) with a lot of money to spend. It is estimated that of the $154 million that philanthropic foundations gave to medical education between 1902 and 1934, the GEB alone was responsible for $90 million. An additional $450 million came from other non-foundation sources during the same time period.
2 Abraham Flexner not only wrote a report criticizing medical education, he also was selected to implement the transformation of the medical educational system he had just studied. While what was implemented was not exactly the same as what had been initially outlined in the report, the continuity provided by Flexner was a tremendous asset to its success.
3 The report was written in close collaboration—indeed collusion—with the predominant professional organization of the time (the American Medical Association).
4 Medical education in 1910 was in an extremely underdeveloped state. The level of capital investment was minimal and the

A System of Scientific Medicine

established institutions had only marginal economic power or significance. As proprietary medical schools were not the most profitable of investments and were subject to prevailing economic swings, there was little desire on the part of the owners to fight to keep the system as it was. Because there was so little resistance to change, the drastic changes were much easier to accomplish.

5 There was a spurious, but quite evident correlation between the changes that occurred in medical education and the improvement of health status in the United States. This seeming relationship abetted support for further changes in medical education.

This ensemble of propitious factors has not existed for any other group trying to enact changes on the scale of those instituted in the wake of the Flexner Report, certainly not in so short a time period.

This book documents the events that led to the Flexner Report and the role that the large philanthropic foundations played in both initiating the study of medical education and in providing the funding to implement the recommendations. The larger plan of the foundations to restructure the medical care system is also documented. Despite the clearly dominant role that the Rockefeller philanthropies played in the transition from a sectarian to a scientific medical education system, it is surprising that only E. Richard Brown, in his 1979 book entitled *Rockefeller Medicine Men*, has specifically told this story.

Although there were other philanthropic foundations who had some interest in medical care, medical education and medical research in the first third of the twentieth century, only the GEB and, to a lesser extent, the Carnegie Foundation were truly significant forces in shaping policy. They were not only the largest foundations but they were also concerned with establishing new policies and expanding the horizons of current approaches to policy development. Most significant of all, the two gave the vast majority of the foundation money that went into medical education and medical research. It is worth noting that restricting this inquiry to the medical education and medical research activities of these

Introduction

foundations ignores their contributions to such fields as public health, psychiatry, life sciences outside of medical school, and medical missionary work in international settings.

This book will show that:

1 The philanthropic foundations were responsible for the major changes in medical research and medical education that occurred in the beginning of the twentieth century.
2 The actions that foundations took were more heavily influenced by the staff of the foundation than by the founders. Frederick T. Gates (not John D. Rockefeller, Sr.) and Henry S. Pritchett (not Andrew Carnegie) were actually responsible for the actions that were taken in the founders' names.
3 Abraham Flexner actually wrote two reports on medical education, one in 1910 and an unpublished one in 1911. Flexner spent from 1911 through 1928 implementing the recommendations of the second report under the auspices of the GEB.
4 It was the unitary focus on medical research on the part of Frederick T. Gates, and his ability to secure large amounts of money from John D. Rockefeller, Sr. that was largely responsible for the research focus that American medical education adopted and still maintains.
5 The differences between the objective conditions of medical education and medical research in the late twentieth century and at the time of the Flexner Report, make it unlikely that a 'Flexner Report' or a total restructuring and redirection within the field of medicine could be implemented today.

The book begins with a brief history of the evolution of foundations in the United States and a description of the development of higher education. A chapter on the attempted merger of Rush Medical College with the University of Chicago explains how the Rockefeller philanthropies first became interested in scientific medicine. The establishment and expansion of the GEB and the role of Gates in the Rockefeller organization is also documented. The development of the first privately endowed research institute in the United States, the Rockefeller Institute, is explored in great detail and the connections between medical research and medical education are examined. The book then shifts to the Carnegie

A System of Scientific Medicine

Foundation to explain the genesis of the Flexner Report of 1910. Several chapters are devoted to explaining the Report and its popular and professional reception. Flexner's later work on the full-time clinical plan on behalf of the GEB rounds out the book.

Frederick T. Gates had a vision of a system of scientific medicine. This volume documents how he orchestrated the role of philanthropic foundations in changing the direction of the field of medical education.

1
From Philanthropy to Foundations

Early American philanthropy is generally associated with the Puritan religion that colonists brought with them from England as part of their heritage. Indeed, before the Revolutionary War the great majority of philanthropy in this country was supplied by the British (Sears 1922:51). After independence, virtually all this aid ceased and American religious organizations and individuals took over the burden of philanthropy. Particularly notable in this regard was Cotton Mather, whose book, *Essays to Do Good* (1710) was a guide to worthy giving whose principles were followed by many Americans, including Benjamin Franklin (Weaver 1967:21). With the gradual acquisition of large amounts of wealth, a change began to overtake American philanthropy. 'Philanthropy', which has been defined by Sears as 'all gifts except those from the State' (Sears 1922:10), was largely replaced by philanthropic foundations, organizations or institutions established by endowment with provisions for future welfare. The earliest of these new philanthropic foundations was the Smithsonian Institution, established in 1846 with $500,000 by James Smithson, an English inventor and scientist (Weaver 1967:24). However the Smithsonian was primarily a research institution and was not directly concerned with welfare (Bremner 1960:53).

The first modern foundation explicitly established to devote itself to human welfare was the Peabody Fund, endowed by George Peabody in 1867 (Morison 1964:IIII). Peabody was a Massachusetts merchant banker who had made his fortune in Baltimore by selling southern cotton to England and importing European luxury goods into the South. His intentions in setting up the Fund are best summarized in his letter of empowerment to the Board of Trustees:

> "I give to you ... the sum of one million dollars, to be by you and your successors held in trust, and the income thereof used and applied, in your discretion, for the promotion and encouragement of intellectual, moral or industrial education among the young of the more destitute portion of the Southern and Southwestern States of our Union, my purpose being that the benefits intended shall be distributed among the entire population, without other distinction than to their needs and opportunities of usefulness to them." [Cleaver 1975:120]

The Fund gave away $3,650,556 between 1868 and 1914 (Sears 1922:90). The Peabody Fund was successful on two levels. First, it fostered ties of cooperation between northern businessmen and southern aristocrats by having them serve together on the same board of trustees. Second, it supported and helped to popularize public schooling for both blacks and whites in the South (Cleaver 1975:120). Dr Barnas Sears, the first director of the fund, used the money to build schools—schools later taken over and supported by southern state governments. After building the schools, he used the Fund to begin training teachers for the schools. The Fund revamped the University of Nashville into the Peabody Normal College in 1875 to foster this goal (Sears 1922:89). It is significant that other northern capitalists also were interested in setting up schools for training teachers of southern youth. In 1867 the Hampton Normal and Agricultural Institute for Negro Education was established by Samuel Armstrong (an ex-Union general) and Robert C. Ogden, the partner of Philadelphia merchant John Wannamaker. This same pair later set up the Tuskeegee Institute with Booker T. Washington as its head, patterned after Hampton (Cleaver 1975:121).

The second modern foundation was the John F. Slater Fund for the Education of Freedmen, established in March 1882 with a gift of $1 million from John F. Slater, a textile manufacturer

From Philanthropy to Foundations

from Connecticut (Cleaver 1975:125). Slater, in his letter of gift, noted that it was the example of the Peabody Fund that he was following when he gave the money to be used primarily for the training of teachers for 'the uplifting of the lately emancipated population of the Southern States and their posterity' (Sears 1922:83).

As Leavell (1930:64) has noted, the assistance given to public education was mainly for the 'establishment and maintenance of industrial and vocational training.' J.L.M. Curry, who became the general agent for both the Peabody and Slater funds in 1891, was an ardent spokesman and advocate for industrial training, proclaiming education as a vital prerequisite for the expansion of northern capital into the South. William Baldwin, who served as a trustee of the Peabody Fund:

> " . . . went South as a businessman conscious of the value of Negro labor. He considered this labor necessary to the efficient operation of his railroad, for he needed thousands of Negro workers—but he needed them trained. He was convinced that the prosperity of the South, as well as his railroad, depended on the productive ability of the population and he felt that the source of this ability was and always would be the Negro." [Bullock 1967:100–01]

Despite this, Leavell noted that 'colored schools were given only two-thirds of the money that was given to white schools' (1930:86). An explanation for this differential giving may be found in an address given by Henry St George Tucker, President of Washington and Lee University, who told a group of northern philanthropists:

> "If it is your idea to educate the Negro, you must have the white of the South with you. If the poor white sees the son of a Negro neighbor enjoying through your munificence benefits denied to his boy, it raises in him a feeling that will render futile all your work. You must lift up the 'poor white' and the Negro together if you would approach success." [*New York World*, April 25, 1901; cited in Fosdick 1962:7]

This endorsement of education in the South was only a part of the overall endorsement of education by capitalists and industrialists throughout the country at this time.

The changing political economy of the United States—1860–1900

The large foundations formed after the turn of the century differed from the earlier foundations both in terms of size and intent. They were not mere evolutionary successors to the smaller foundations, but rather the historically specific reflections of the objective conditions and needs of the political economy in the period around the turn of the century. A brief overview of the major changes is presented below:

1 *Population:* The most noticeable change in the United States during this period was the tremendous increase in population —from 23,261,000 in 1850 to 76,094,000 in 1900 and to 92,407,000 in 1910 (US Bureau of the Census 1960:7). Between 1850 and 1900, 16 million immigrants entered the country, with the majority settling in the Northeast (US Bureau of the Census 1960:57). Because so many of the immigrants were children, by 1900, 53 per cent of the population was under the age of twenty-four (US Bureau of the Census 1960:8).
2 *Urbanization:* In 1860, less than 15 per cent of the country lived in towns with populations over 8,000. By 1900, over one-third of the population did. Between 1860 and 1910, 11,826,000 people moved into urban areas; immigrants accounted for 41 per cent of this increase (Spring 1973:3). The populations of urban areas increased rapidly. New York, which had less than 700,000 in 1850, had over 3 million by 1900, and Chicago which had less than 100,000 population in 1850, had over a million by 1900 (Beard and Beard 1937:206). The increasing urbanization led to changes in the mode of living as well. By 1900, over 90 per cent of the populace of Manhattan lived in rented homes or tenements and over 80 per cent of the populations of Boston, Fall River, Jersey City and Memphis lived similarly. Detroit, at the head of the list of cities with mortgage-free homes, had only 20 per cent (Beard and Beard 1937:207).
3 *Industrialization:* In 1860, the capital invested in manufacturing was slightly over $1 billion, and 1,500,000 industrial workers were employed. By 1900 capital investment had risen to over $12 billion and the workforce had increased to 5½ million (Beard

and Beard 1937:176). By 1900, over 75 per cent of manufactured goods came from enterprises organized along corporate lines. The average annual Gross National Product (GNP) for 1890 –93 of $13.5 billion had increased to $24.2 billion for 1902–06, an increase in per capita GNP from $210 to $294 (US Bureau of the Census 1960:139). The national wealth of the United States had increased from one-third of that of the United Kingdom in 1850 to over $13 billion larger than the United Kingdom's $52 billion in 1900. In his book *Triumphant Democracy*, Andrew Carnegie said: "The sixty-five million Americans of today could buy up the one hundred and forty millions of Russians, Austrians and Spaniards, or, after purchasing wealthy France, would have pocket money to acquire Denmark, Norway, Switzerland and Greece" (Beard and Beard 1937:205).

4 *Labor:* Large-scale labor violence and organized trade union activity started after 1875 with the emergence of a large industrial proletariat. The Haymarket Massacre of 1886, the Homestead Strike of 1892, the Pullman Strike of 1894, Coxey's Army of 1894 and the formation of socialist-syndicalist trade or industrial unions (e.g., the Industrial Workers of the World in 1905), were only the tip of the iceberg of labor discontent (Adamic 1931). Labor discontent was not restricted to industrial workers. The populist movement had crystallized into a genuine political threat to the existing two-party system and had put fifteen members into Congress by 1900 (Pollack 1966). The Granges and Farmers' Associations played a similar role to that of the unions in rural and farm areas (Wasserman 1972).

5 *Wealth:* A newspaper survey in 1892 revealed the presence of 4,047 millionaires in the United States. A 1902 almanac survey estimated the number at 3,561 (Ratner 1953). More important than the absolute number of millionaires was the size of the larger fortunes. John D. Rockefeller, Sr. had a reported annual income of $40 million and his total wealth at the turn of the century was in the area of $200 million (Nevins 1940). Andrew Carnegie sold his interest in the Carnegie Steel Corporation to United States Steel for $495 million (Wall 1970:803). Contrasted with this extreme of wealth was an increase in poverty at the other end of the scale. While subsistence conditions were

the norm in rural areas, the cities were inundated with unemployed and unemployable immigrants from both abroad and from rural areas.

In summary, the changes that can be most easily noted about this time period are: 1) an increasing population; primarily urban-based; 2) large numbers of immigrants; 3) increasing industrialization; 4) increasing wealth and poverty. Certain other changes were important to the creation of philanthropic foundations:

1 In certain industries (primarily oil, heavy metals, and related transportation industries) accumulation was proceeding at a pace so great that the normal recirculation mechanisms were inadequate to safely recycle the profits that were being generated. The dilemma faced by John D. Rockefeller, Sr. for example was how to reinvest oil profits ("petro-dollars") in the face of social and political limitations on total reinvestment of the money and the problems posed by siphoning this money out of the system through hoarding. This is perhaps the meaning of Frederick T. Gates's warning to the elder Rockefeller: "Your fortune is rolling up, rolling up like an avalanche! You must distribute it faster than it grows! If you do not it will crush you, and your children, and your children's children" (Nevins 1940: 291).

Simple recirculation of the profits by reinvestment in either land or new industrial ventures, as well as investment of the money in overseas markets, was all being carried out by the Rockefeller office. There were political and social restrictions, however, on the amount of profit that could be recycled in this manner. The early legal battles of the Standard Oil Trust in the 1890s and the passage of early anti-trust laws in that same period, as well as the threatened tax on incomes, all seemed to impose clear limits on the absolute total wealth that could be accrued by the individual entrepreneur. Hoarding of the profits was a potential threat to stagnate the economy. Thus there was a need to do something with the money but clear limits on what could be done.

2 The level of class struggle seemed to be on the increase. Not only were labor agitation and unionization rampant, but the

European immigrants were bringing socialist ideas and concepts with them. A high percentage of the people now employed in industry were formerly agrarians or petty-commodity producers and they had to learn capitalist time horizons and work norms. Along with the breakdown of the traditional social control mechanisms, which occurred with the shift from Europe to America and from farm to city, came the need to find a new mechanism to ensure social order. Since the Civil War had come the development of education—both secondary education to teach work discipline and skills to working-class people, and higher education to prepare a middle-class elite to administer the new social order. The de-skilling of heavy industry after the 1890s and the concurrent attempts at labor market stratification with the rise of professionals, managers, and technicians also necessitated a new educational system (Brody 1969). Thus, at the turn of the century, there was a need for investment in those areas of society which would help ensure a more stable and productive workforce—education, welfare, medical care.

3 The subjective factors, by definition, differ for each of the large fortunes. In the case of Carnegie, with no son to whom he might leave his fortune and an inordinate desire to be "loved", giving the money away seemed to be the only way to rid himself of his fortune. Rockefeller, who was deeply religious, had always believed in charity and did not want to die disgraced. Neither he nor Carnegie was profligate (although Carnegie was somewhat more extravagant than Rockefeller) and that removed another avenue for surplus reduction.

As capitalists, neither of these men, nor any of the other wealthy men who set up foundations in this period, would dream of just giving away money. They needed to create a rationale that would justify the distribution of their fortunes. The most prominent example of this came in the "Gospel of Wealth".

The Gospel of Wealth

The Gospel of Wealth has become a catch-word for the interpretation of the reasons behind the formation of the large-scale philanthropic ventures around the turn of the century. In the June and December 1889 issues of the *North American Review*, there appeared an essay by Andrew Carnegie entitled "Wealth". The essay received wide attention being called "the finest article I have ever published in the Review" by editor Allen Thorndike Rice (Wall 1970: 806). The essay was reprinted in Britain in the *Pall Mall Gazette* under the title "The Gospel of Wealth". The essay was also reprinted in 1900 along with other essays by Carnegie in a book that received mass circulation.

The thesis of the article came from the first line of the essay: "The problem of our age is the proper administration of wealth; that the ties of brotherhood may still bind together the rich and poor in harmonious relationship" (Carnegie 1962:14). Carnegie limited his argument to a discussion of philanthropy under capitalism, assuming away the possibility of an alternative economic mode through the use of the following argument:

> "Objections to the foundations upon which society is based are not in order, because the condition of the race is better with these than it has been with any other which has been tried. Of the effect of any substitutes proposed we cannot be sure. The Socialist or Anarchist who seeks to overturn present conditions is to be regarded as attacking the foundation upon which civilization itself rests, for civilization took its start from the day when the capable, industrious workman said to his incompetent and lazy fellow, 'if thou dost not sow, thou shalt not reap,' and thus ended primitive Communism by separating the drones from the bees. One who studies this subject will soon be brought face to face with the conclusion that upon the sacredness of property civilization itself depends—the right of the laborer to his hundred dollars in the savings bank, and equally the legal right of the millionaire to his millions. Every man must be allowed 'to sit under his own vine and fig tree, with none to make afraid,' if human society is to advance, or even remain so far advanced as it is. To those who propose to substitute Communism for this intense Individualism, the answer therefore is: the race has tried that. All progress from that barbarous day to the present time has resulted from its displacement." [Carnegie 1962:17]

Carnegie considered three possible alternatives for the disposal of surplus wealth. The individual can either leave his wealth to his family, bequeath it for public purposes or administer it during his lifetime for public benefit. Carnegie argued that leaving it to one's family was the least desirable of the three because of the problems of inherited wealth. The article is full of proverbs and homilies regarding the inappropriateness of inherited wealth. According to Carnegie the second alternative was better, but in leaving a fortune for public purposes, one often finds that the goals one hoped to accomplish are thwarted by greedy and jealous heirs. The third alternative was thus the only acceptable one:

> "There remains, then, but one mode of using great fortunes; but in this we have the true antidote for the temporary unequal distribution of wealth, the reconciliation of the rich and the poor—a reign of harmony, another ideal, differing, indeed, from that of the Communist in requiring only the further evolution of existing conditions, not the total overthrow of our civilization. It is founded upon the present most intense Individualism, and the race is prepared to put it in practice by degrees whenever it pleases. Under its sway we shall have an ideal State, in which the surplus wealth of the few will become, in the best sense, the property of the many, because administered for the common good; and this wealth, passing through the hands of the few, can be made a much more potent force for the evolution of our race than if distributed in small sums to the people themselves. Even the poorest can be made to see this, and to agree that great sums gathered by some of their fellow citizens and spent for public purposes, from which the masses reap the principal benefit, are more valuable to them than if scattered among themselves in trifling amounts through the course of many years." [Carnegie 1962:23]

Carnegie devoted the rest of his article to enumerating the seven fields worthy of philanthropic support. They are: 1) founding a university "a noble use of wealth" (Carnegie 1962: 33)—Carnegie pointed out that only the very wealthy can do this and mentioned such names as Johns Hopkins, Ezra Cornell, Leland Stanford —men who had already established major universities; 2) a free library, Carnegie's own favorite benefaction; 3) the founding or extension of hospitals, medical colleges, laboratories and other institutions connected with the alleviation of human suffering, and especially with the prevention, rather than the cure, of human ills; 4) public parks; 5) concert and meeting halls; 6) swimming pools and baths; 7) churches.

The reviews of Carnegie's 'gospel' were generally, though not unanimously, favorable. People had specific grudges against the order in which the fields of beneficence were listed. Ministers and mission boards were particularly enraged at being placed last, even after swimming pools and baths. In addition, many people thought that other categories could have been included such as artists, writers, musicians, orphanages, private schools, and so on. A British magazine, *The Nineteenth Century*, published a symposium entitled "Irresponsible Wealth" with statements by the three leading religious figures of Britain, the Archbishop of Westminster, the Chief Rabbi and a noted Methodist minister. The Archbishop and the Rabbi pointed out, amid general praise for Mr. Carnegie, that nothing in the article could not be found in the mainstreams of Judeo–Christian tradition. The minister was much more critical, noting that Carnegie did not deal with the fundamental issue of society—the distribution of wealth, but chose instead to deal with the lesser issue of its administration. He went on to add that in a truly Christian society there would be no millionaires, that millionaires were themselves a symbol of man's fall from grace. He concluded by saying that if Carnegie's gospel were not quickly adopted and if the growing gulf between rich and poor did not stop, then a terrible social upheaval would result:

> "In London we are living on the verge of a volcano.... Never, since the downfall of the Roman Empire and the dissolution of the ancient world, has Europe witnessed so perilous a situation as exists in London today. Never has there been so vast a multitude of half-starved men, within sight of boundless wealth, and outside the control of the Christian church." [Wall 1970: 810]

A more sophisticated critical view of the gospel was offered by William Jewet Tucker, a Professor of Religion at Andover Seminary, later to become President of Dartmouth College. In a review written for the *Andover Review* of June 1891, Tucker critiques Carnegie's gospel:

> "It is especially significant for what has been discussed. With a single exception, the discussion has been confined to the question of the

From Philanthropy to Foundations

charitable disposition of private wealth, without entering at all, except in the way of illustration, upon the more serious question of the vast concentration of wealth in private hands. ... If he is to preach this gospel of wealth to the rich, he must above all things make them feel the 'inevitableness' of their lot. They must be made to realize that they are the necessary product of the system to which they belong. There must needs be the very rich; if not these, then others. Some persons cannot escape the responsibility of riches, however great at times may seem to them the 'advantages of poverty'. The inevitable factor in society is not so certainly the poor as the rich. The rich ye have with you always. ... While [Mr Carnegie] is asking. ... this question about the disposal of the vast surplus of private wealth, society is taking hold in very serious fashion of the other end of the problem, and asking why there should be such a vast surplus of private wealth. ... I can conceive of no greater mistake, more monstrous in the end to religion if not to society, than that of trying to make charity do the work of justice."

Tucker then delineated the question-begging aspects of Carnegie's thesis:

"The question is not, how shall private wealth be returned to the public? but, why should it exist in such bewildering amounts? Mr. Carnegie's gospel is really a belated gospel. It comes too late for a social remedy. What it does accomplish is to call attention to the fact of the enormous surplus of private wealth. The honest and courageous endeavour of a millionaire to return his fortune to society, and his call to his fellow-millionaires to do likewise, brings them, as a class, before the public, and puts the public upon a reckoning of the volume of wealth in their hands. Consciously or unconsciously, Mr. Carnegie has hit upon the great object-lesson in our economic civilization. It is not pauperism, conspicuous and grievous as that is, but the concentration of wealth. The most striking, and in many ways the most startling, feature of the economic situation is, not that the poor are growing poorer, ... but that the rich are becoming so very rich."

Tucker concluded his review with the following:

"My criticism of Mr. Carnegie's scheme has been that, to the degree in which it is organized and made the ruling method of adjusting wealth to society it becomes a vast system of patronage, than which nothing can in the final issue create a more hopeless social condition. And further, that the assumption on which it rests, that wealth is the inevitable possession of the few, and is best administered by them for the many, begs the whole question of economic justice now before society, and relegates it to the field of charity. ... I would hinder no man's gifts in the largest charity; I would withhold no honour from the giver; but I would accept no amount of charity as a measure of the present social need, or in settlement of the present economic demand." [Tucker 1891: 631-45]

In his definitive biography of Carnegie, Wall found no evidence that Carnegie was aware of this review. He noted that Carnegie had found in his gospel a justification for his life that was entirely satisfying and was therefore not likely to change his views in any respects (Wall 1970: 815).

In February, 1893 in the *Review of Reviews*, American edition, an article appeared entitled "American Millionaires and Their Public Gifts". It was unsigned but is attributed to Albert Shaw, the editor of the *Review*. The article purported to survey the field of philanthropy and see if America's wealthy were living up to Mr. Carnegie's gospel and distributing their wealth in their lifetime. Men of knowledge and influence in the large cities of the country were asked to rate the beneficence of their local millionaires according to the criteria set up by Carnegie. A similar survey was done in the same journal in 1904 (Curti, Green, and Nash 1963: 416-35). This indicates that the gospel of wealth became an important justification for the growth of philanthropy on the philanthropists' own terms. Rockefeller, Sr. is said to have written Carnegie an enthusiastic letter of congratulations for his gospel, telling him to: "be assured, your example will bear fruits" (Weaver 1967: 35).

2
The Growth of Higher Education in the United States

Higher education in the United States went through a period of dramatic reform between 1860 and 1910. This period marked changes in educational form as well as content. The seeds for this reform had been sown earlier and to perceptive observers the writing was on the wall as early as the 1840s. Carnoy (1974) and Katz (1968) show how the first of these reforms started with the development of the secondary school in the 1840s. At that time, primary education was solely the concern of local groups each autonomous from control or coordination. The concept of the public secondary school was developed by educational reformers who, like Horace Mann, worked in northeastern states that were undergoing rapid industrialization at the time and needed differently trained workers. By its very nature, the school would cross local boundaries necessitating centralized control and coordination. Under the influence if not the control of the reformers, the high schools soon became more practically oriented so as to better meet the needs of the growing industrial class. These changes in the high school were soon felt in the college. In 1842 Francis Wayland, the President of Brown University, said in a famous and prophetic report: "If the colleges did not provide the training desired by the mercantile and industrial interests ... businessmen would set up competing schools" (Hofstadter and Hardy 1952: 23–4). Carnoy (1974: 236) described the reasons why businessmen needed a new school:

A System of Scientific Medicine

> "Thus the Movement for public education in the United States began [in the 1840s and 1850s] in the industrializing northern states under pressure from reformers who represented the views of a growing bourgeoisie. Local industrialists saw schooling as a means to offset the disruptive social conditions of factory life; some institution was necessary to provide the moral guidance and control which the family and church had supplied in precapitalist society. The South didn't participate in this movement until northern capital took control of its institutions. Public education as it developed in the United States was the reformers' answer to the growth of industry and the crisis it caused in the traditional social structure. Schooling was seen by the reformers and industrialists alike as promoting their common vision of an ordered and purposeful and progressive society. In conjunction with this view, it also helped to preserve class structure in the face of economic and social change."

One of the first issues of reform in higher education during the 1860s was the adoption of the elective system. The elective system, which did away with required course work and allowed the student to specialize in a field, was first instituted by Charles Eliot at Harvard. It was not long before most colleges in the country adopted the elective system. Hofstadter and Hardy (1952: 50) noted that:

> "The elective system seemed like an academic transcription of liberal capitalist thinking. It added to the total efficiency of society by conforming to the principle of division of intellectual labor. It was pluralistic, in the sense that it recognized spontaneous differences in individual interests ..."

The elective system was the first step in a larger campaign of transformation of the college. Curti and Nash (cited in Smith 1974: 67, 72) pointed out:

> "Increasingly, the men of means were businessmen who built railroads, extended commercial networks and directed the operations of factories ... instead of patronizing the classical colleges run by and for the old elite, many nineteenth century entrepreneurs sought to transform existing institutions or to found new ones that would be more responsive to current demands as *they* defined them. The great fortunes of the members of the new elite gave them the opportunity, through philanthropy, to implement their novel educa-

tional ideas ... Their common experience in the world of business and industry impressed upon them the need for technical talent. They were well aware that the graduates coming from the campuses of the classical colleges were totally unprepared to meet the problems involved in building a bridge, operating a bank or designing a machine."

Engineering and the sciences were particularly undeveloped in the United States in the first half of the nineteenth century. West Point, the United States Military Academy set up in 1802 by Congress, served as the first technical institute in the United States (Rudolph 1962: 228). Rennssalear Polytechnical Institute in Troy, New York, which was established in 1824, was the leading producer of engineers in the United States until the Civil War (Rudolph 1962: 229). In 1847 a $50,000 benefaction was given to Harvard University by Abbott Lawrence for scientific education. The Lawrence School, as it was called, became the first undergraduate program in the United States to grant a bachelor of science degree (first granted in 1851). Although Lawrence had intended this benefaction to support the growth of engineering, a member of the faculty (Louis Agassiz) and the President of the University steered the school toward comparative zoology instead (Rudolph 1962: 231–32). At Yale University, a school of applied chemistry was set up in 1847 and a program of civil engineering was added in 1852. In 1860 with a gift of $100,000 from Joseph Sheffield, this school became the Sheffield Scientific School (Rudolph 1962: 232). What is most important about these early developments in scientific education is that these schools were the learning centers of the men who would go on to create a new generation of scientifically oriented universities—Charles Eliot at the Lawrence School and Daniel Coit Gilman at the Sheffield School. The former was responsible for the new directions at Harvard while the latter was the first President of the Johns Hopkins University. In 1851, Dartmouth, Rochester, Denison, Michigan, Illinois, University of North Carolina, New York University, Iowa, and Missouri all started departments of science (Rudolph 1962: 233). Between 1860 and 1870 more than twenty-five other institutions opened such departments.

After the Civil War a new breed of college emerged in the

A System of Scientific Medicine

United States. Dedicated to science and technology, schools such as the Massachusetts Institute of Technology, Cornell University, Lehigh University and Lafayette College were opened (Rudolph 1962: 246). The first graduate degree, the doctor of philosophy, was awarded by Yale in 1861 (Rudolph 1962: 269). Graduate schools began to proliferate on the American scene in the 1870s and 1880s with Johns Hopkins in 1876, Columbia in 1880, Michigan in 1881, Clark University and Catholic University in 1889, Harvard in 1890, and Vanderbilt, Chicago, Wisconsin, Michigan State, Nebraska, and Kansas in the 1890s. The new institution was of increasing importance as is indicated by the fact that in 1926, fifty years after its founding, 1,000 of Johns Hopkins' 1,400 graduates were on college and university faculties in the United States (Rudolph 1962: 335–36). Hofstadter and Hardy (1952: 57–8) pointed out that:

"Since the emergence of the university coincided with the period of industrialism, corporate business, urbanism, growing social complexity, and the advancement of heightening prestige of science, the new graduate and professional schools that proliferated ... were naturally molded by these developments. ... The attempt to be 'scientific' therefore spread from the sciences themselves into every sphere of intellectual life. Law schools tried to teach 'scientific law', historians to write 'scientific' history and even classicists, trying to be scientific, turned to philology. That excessive scientism which has become one of the banes of modern American culture may have had its roots far back in the nation's past; but there can be no doubt that it was unanimously quickened between 1860 and 1900."

Alongside the growing number of graduate schools with their emphasis on science and technology came professional schools also attuned to the needs of the times. Schools of business and commerce were started at the University of Pennsylvania in 1881, Chicago in 1898, New York University in 1900, Dartmouth in 1900 and Harvard in 1908, the last being endowed with $5 million by the banker George Baker (Curti and Nash 1965: 74–5). Between 1912 and 1920 MIT received $20 million from George Eastman, the founder of Kodak, who noticed that a large number of his best employees came from that school (Curti and Nash 1965: 78–80). The Stevens family, who were inventors and mechanics, established the Stevens

Institute of Technology in Hoboken, New Jersey, in 1867. The school contained the first department of mechanical engineering in the United States (Curti and Nash 1965: 78–80).

Virtually every school found its own patron or patrons to support and uplift it. Columbia University had among its donors Morgan, Vanderbilt, Cutting, Havemeyer, Pulitzer, Schermerhorn, Schiff, Fish, and even its own President Low. New York University had the financier Jay Gould; Chicago and Brown had John D. Rockefeller, Sr.; Kenyon College had Marc Hanna; Rochester and MIT had George Eastman and Rennssalear Polytechnical Institute had Mrs. Russell Sage (Rudolph 1962: 426). Between 1878 and 1898, approximately $140 million was given to educational institutions by individuals. Between 1750 and 1850 only 174 colleges were formed in the United States; between 1850 and 1900, 453 were established. In 1870 there were 67,530 students enrolled in institutions of higher learning; by 1890 this number had increased to 156,756 and by 1910 to 355,212 (Smith 1974: 73). It is important to note though that college was still restricted to the small minority that could afford it. The percentage of Americans of college age attending college rose from 4.01 per cent in 1900 to only 4.84 per cent in 1910 (Veysey 1965: 2).

This support for higher education by wealthy industrialists and financiers led to changes in the nature of the educational venture. Hofstadter and Metzger (1955: 414) noted that:

"Inevitably, the increase in the size of the gifts changed the relations of donor to recipient. Borrowing a term from economic history, one may say that the givers became entrepreneurs in the field of higher education. They took the initiative in providing funds and deciding their general purposes. William Rainey Harper [President of the University of Chicago] wrote in 1905 that 'in the case of 90 per cent of the money given to a large institution the initiative is taken by the donor, and not by the university concerned.' This was a reversal of the procedure that had been in effect before the Civil War, when college presidents sued for alms on the basis of needs which they determined. But passive roles did not suit the new men of wealth. ... It was (to take a crowning example) Andrew Carnegie who decided to give retirement pensions to professors, and this without their prior solicitation."

A System of Scientific Medicine

Where did the idea to support higher education come from? Clearly it was not just the needs of the economic system which led to this great infusion of capital into education, although this was certainly an important aspect of the process. As Cremin (1964:59) noted in his *Transformation of the School*:

> "To look on the Nineties is to sense an awakening of social conscience, a growing belief that this incredible suffering was neither the fault nor the inevitable lot of the sufferers, that it could certainly be alleviated, and that the road to alleviation was neither charity nor revolution, but in the last analysis education."

Cremin concluded that it was educational reformers and social scientists like Lester Ward and Albion Small who did much to promote the idea that education would allay class violence:

> " . . . [Lester F.] Ward, unlike Spencer and Sumner, conceived of education as the foremost activity of mankind, the 'great panacea' for all social ills. Following Auguste Comte he argued that social salvation lay in a vast diffusion of information, especially scientific information, among the citizenry at large. The popularization of knowledge would inevitably create widespread understanding of man's relations with nature; this, in turn, would enable men in their daily lives to harmonize natural phenomena with human advantage; and this, ultimately, would lead to the greatest happiness for the greatest number. Education that was scientific, popular and universal could be the 'mainspring of progress', the 'piston of civilization', the 'embodiment of all that is progressive.'" [Cremin 1964:97]

Education was looked upon as the primary means of socializing the heterogeneous grouping that America had become. What is most interesting though is the shape that this education took. The educational division of labor was remarkably similar to the industrial division of labor. The elective system led to the division of academic labor into departments which expanded to form graduate schools as vertical extensions for further research and specialization. This was exactly the pattern of labor division that had occurred with the generation of large-scale capitalist enterprise and was closely followed by the development of medicine as one branch of this higher education.

The abundance of philanthropy pouring into education led to

an anarchic situation. Individual philanthropists gave to their favorite institutions without regard for need, duplication of facilities and equipment, location of institutions, competition, ability of institutions to draw students, or any other factor. This situation was analogous to the market-place anarchy prevalent in industry in pre-trust days. The situation in educational philanthropy was thus in clear contradiction to the efforts of these same philanthropists in their business lives who conspired to control production and market prices. This contradiction between the individual philanthropist and the collective capitalist was attenuated by the creation of large-scale foundations for educational philanthropy. Foundations acted not so much as charitable organizations as coordinators of educational philanthropy. Foundations would decide what schools to support and how to support them, which institutions should grow and which should wither away. In short, foundations controlled the development of higher education in the United States.

Just as the concentrated development of higher education led to the specialization into professional and graduate schools, the development of educational foundations led to their specialization into fields of support as well. There were different strategies for accomplishing this purpose as can be seen by the differing strategies formulated by the two largest foundations. The Rockefeller GEB attempted to transform the field by giving large sums of money to specially selected schools. It assumed that schools which did not receive money would be forced to reorient themselves in the desired direction. The Carnegie Foundation for the Advancement of Teaching attacked the problem through a form of certification, weeding out those colleges which did not meet their specifications. This same dynamic was evident in medical education with the Rockefeller philanthropies supporting good schools and the Carnegie philanthropies trying to eliminate bad schools.

With the preceding as a general overview of the changes taking place in both philanthropy and education, we now proceed to look at the development of the Rockefeller General Education Board, the first of the major educational philanthropies and also a major contributor to medical education.

3
Frederick T. Gates and the General Education Board

Frederick T. Gates was born on July 2, 1853 in rural Broome County, New York. His father was a Baptist minister who worked in the poor parishes of south central New York. When he was fourteen, the Gates family moved to Highland, Kansas. In 1873, aged twenty, Gates prepared to enter the University of Rochester in Rochester, New York. He found, though, that he could save money by studying at home for two years. In 1875 he formally entered the university from which he graduated in 1877.

In 1877, upon graduation, Gates enrolled in the Rochester Theological Seminary in a three-year course that would lead to his ordination as a Baptist minister. In the spring of 1880, he received an invitation to become the pastor of the Fifth Avenue Baptist Church of Minneapolis, Minnesota, having been recommended for the post by the President of the Seminary, Dr. Strong. The pastorate was small and poor with little chance of future growth. Nevertheless Gates was able to convince the church elders to build a new and larger church in a better section of Minneapolis. He was also to marry Lucia Fowler Perkins in 1882, a young woman he had met while a student in Rochester. Lucia died suddenly from an internal ailment on October 31, 1883. In 1886, Gates took another wife, Emma Lucille Cahoon of Racine, Wisconsin. While the new church was an improvement on the older one, it was still overshadowed by the other Baptist church in Minneapolis. As Gates began to realize how limited his pastorate was, he became more involved in statewide educational work in Minnesota. Through this work he came to know Mr. George Pillsbury, founder of Pillsbury Flour Company, one of the richest Baptists in the mid-west. Pillsbury was a congregant at the other Minneapolis church but saw a lot of potential in young Gates. He wanted to endow a Baptist academy in Minnesota and was impressed by the sage advice offered by Gates. Gates was selected by Pillsbury to head up the canvassing effort around the state to raise money for the new school. Gates's unequivocal success in raising money began to bring him national attention in Baptist educational circles. He was elected secretary of the American Baptist Education Society (ABES), a national fund-raising group.

It was in this context that Gates first came into contact with John D. Rockefeller regarding the creation of what was to become the University of Chicago. In September, 1891, Gates accepted an offer from Rockefeller to join him and take charge of his philanthropic affairs. Gates and his family moved back to the New York area, taking up residence in Montclair, New Jersey.

Gates's initial job was to rationalize the philanthropic giving of Rockefeller. Rockefeller received daily hundreds of letters requesting money and aid from individuals and institutions. Although he was in the process of retiring from active management of the Standard Oil Company, Rockefeller had neither time nor inclination to do the necessary research into whether these requests were genuine or legitimate. Gates's strategy in dealing with this problem consisted of taking Rockefeller out of the business of "retail philanthropy" and installing him in the business of "wholesale philanthropy". For example, Rockefeller received large numbers of requests for aid from the various Baptist parishes of New York and Brooklyn. What Gates did was to establish a central New York agency with staff that would evaluate the individual requests for aid. To this one central body would go a large check, and it would be responsible for doling out smaller amounts to the various requesters who merited largesse. Any letters that came to the Rockefeller office from New York area Baptist churches would simply be routed to this new central agency. Gates set up dozens of these agencies thereby greatly simplifying the logistical task of the Rockefeller office and at the same time freeing himself up to deal with more pressing issues of philanthropic policy.

This application of wholesale philanthropy appealed to Rockefeller who saw in it the same concentration and centralization that had been applied so effectively to the oil industry. He became more and more impressed with Gates and soon asked him to begin to investigate some of his personal investments. Just as Rockefeller was besieged with requests to donate money for various philanthropic efforts, there was no end to the invitations he received to invest in syndicates and other schemes for making money. As Gates began to investigate some of these investment schemes, by traveling around the country, he found that more times than not Rockefeller was being robbed blind. He worked with Rockefeller to either sell out of the unprofitable syndicates or buy up the ones that had potential. In many cases, Gates was put on the Board of Directors or made President of these companies. As Rockefeller began to trust Gates more and more, Gates's responsibilities within the Rockefeller organization increased.

The success that Gates had with wholesale philanthropy in religious charity led him to consider applying this concept to education as well. It was in this context that the plans for a grand philanthropic venture in education began to emerge. The result of these plans was the General Education Board.

The General Education Board

In 1899 the Conference for Southern Education was created as a vehicle to coordinate northern philanthropic educational ventures in the South. The executive committee of the Conference was called the Southern Education Board. In 1901, John D. Rockefeller, Jr. took part in the activities of the Conference and became convinced of the worthiness of the field of education as an outlet for philanthropic investment. The result was the creation of the General Education Board (GEB) in 1902, the first major Rockefeller philanthropy. The GEB received a charter from Congress in 1903. Frederick T. Gates not only was the originator of the GEB but served as the Chairman of its Board from 1907 to

Frederick T. Gates and the General Education Board

1917. His power over the GEB was enormous as was suggested by Gates's assertion in his autobiography: "Up to 1917 when I resigned as chairman, the policies of the Board had been formulated by me, its beneficiaries had been chosen, and the amount and conditions of gifts had been largely influenced by me" (Gates 1977: 218). As a direct descendant of the Southern Education Board, the bulk of its work was concentrated in the South during its early years (Fosdick 1962). Its main accomplishments were the setting up of a system of southern public education and aid to 'negro' public schools, as well as agricultural assistance to southern farmers. On June 3, 1905 Gates wrote a memo to Rockefeller, Sr. in which he advocated the creation of a "great fund for the promotion of a system of higher education in the United States", as well as funds for other activities (Gates Papers, Rockefeller Foundation Archives). Within two weeks of this memo, Rockefeller gave $10 million in endowment to the GEB for that very purpose. The actual history of the gift starts earlier as I will attempt to document.

The nature of the capitalist support to southern education, and negro education as well, can be gleaned from this letter from Gates to Wallace Buttrick in reference to a small gift from Rockefeller, Sr. to a southern negro school: "[Mr. Rockefeller] contributes these little doles from time to time simply to encourage the colored friends in self help and for the sake of securing a certain directive authority over their movements" (Gates Papers, Rockefeller Foundation Archives, June 30, 1901).

Under the competitive threat of an educational foundation being considered by Andrew Carnegie, Gates set to work to beat him to the punch. In a letter dated April 18, 1905, having mentioned that Carnegie was about to start giving money to small colleges in the United States, Gates reflected on the question of what the Rockefellers could do:

> "The Congressional charter of the GEB would perhaps furnish the legal powers desired. The board could be so enlarged and reconstructed as to cover the north as well as the south. The fund could be kept together and made perpetual and if its income could be expended under the guidance of the most enlightened businessmen and educators in the United States, it would do more good in a century than two or three times the amount of money

distributed arbitrarily and at random. . . . the money should be used for such institutions at such locations for such specific purposes and to gain such general ends as will tend to produce in time and always tend toward an ideal system of education from the high schools up to the universities and with no duplication and with every part duly adjusted like a machine to its corresponding part. The whole compact, efficient, economic." [Gates Papers, Rockefeller Family Archives]

Gates discussed this idea with several leading educators and wrote back to Rockefeller, Sr. on April 24, 1905:

"Andrews' [E. Benjamin Andrews, President of Brown University] approval [of a large endowment in the hands of trustees, the income to be used only in colleges] was enthusiastic and unqualifed and he thought it the greatest good that could possibly be done for education in the United States. His objections to the way it was traditionally done were (1) Boards of Trustees were made up of men who know almost nothing of higher education; (2) Presidents of Colleges are usually ministers who also know nothing about higher education; (3) that the colleges can teach Latin, Greek and mathematics but nothing modern; (4) that the distribution is extremely uneven and to give money to these schools is just to perpetuate their influence and not achieve anything . . . if on the other hand we could have a great endowment concentrated in able hands who could keep it intact and perhaps indeed might make it grow. Mr. Morris K. Jessup and Mr. George Foster Peabody, by allowing trust funds which they, as treasurers, control to participate in some of the railroad bond syndicates which they as bankers manage have almost doubled the trust funds put in their hands. Mr. Jessup has added $800,000 to the Peabody Fund by advantageous investment and sharing with his fund some of his syndicate opportunities. Such men can guard funds where ordinary college treasurers and boards of trustees are perfectly helpless. I have seen lists of investments from reputable colleges that almost make me sick. Only a part of the service rendered to the college, and a small part, would be the money annually given. This annual appropriation would be the golden key which would unlock the whole college to the enlightened suggestion of the central Board. A trained corps of auditors sent out by this central Board could gradually adjust the bookkeeping of all colleges to the highest standard and require these standards to be maintained as a condition. The central Board could have an advisory relation with respect to the investments, they could suggest competent and experienced architects who know what is needed for buildings, they could have a bureau which could be of invaluable service in suggesting teachers, professors and presidents. They could, in conjunction with the university presidents, do much towards requiring a uniform system of entrance requirements and proper limitations to the work which should be attempted." [Gates Papers, Rockefeller Family Archives]

Gates had other ideas about the value of this fund and how it could reorganize higher education. On May 22, 1905 he sent a memo to Rockefeller, Sr. including data relating to the size and finances of colleges appealing to the GEB for funds. Gates was impressed by the smaller colleges because they provided for closer relations between the faculty and students and among the students themselves. He continued:

"This is the best possible training for life, but it requires for its fullest development that the student group should be united by close bonds of fellowship and of common interests. I seem to see in the great universities, with the looseness of ties which comes from the obliteration of class lines, and the tendency to the emphasis exclusively on scholarship, a loosening of this most wholesome influence." [Gates Papers, Rockefeller Family Archives]

Gates continued, in a somewhat different vein:

"The establishment of such a great fund as this for these general purposes would be in the line along which the great business interests of the country have been developed, and it would seem particularly fitting that Mr. Rockefeller should be the one to establish such a fund. After sufficient time has elapsed to enable the public to see the business developments of this generation in their proper perspective, I am inclined to think that they will consider Mr. Rockefeller's greatest contribution to the progress of civilization has been the working out and the application to manufacture and commerce of these great principles of consolidation and highly specialized administration which distinguishes the new industry from the old. The very things for which he is now being most severely criticized will prove to be the things on which his lasting and honorable fame will rest."

Following up on this theme of the relation of this new educational philanthropy to the emerging industrial organizational forms was a letter dated June 6, 1905 in which Gates continued:

> "The moral influence of such a board, the possibilities of mutual helpfulness and cooperation which it will introduce among institutions of learning and the economies which it will suggest and secure both in administration and teaching force and the use of men. The ways in which it can select men and direct their energies toward common ends can only be illustrated in my mind successfully by the Standard Oil Company as it is, when compared with what might easily be imagined to be the condition in the oil industry if in its stead the universal competitive system of say 1870 had been continued." [Gates Papers, Rockefeller Family Archives]

Rockefeller was in general agreement with Gates's plan but he had a suggestion which though in line with Gates's ideas about centralization and elimination of competition in industry and education, was absolute anathema to Gates—to go jointly into this venture with Andrew Carnegie. While newspapers of the day tried to show the two industrialists in friendly competition, at least in their battle over who was giving more philanthropy (Corner 1965: 51-2; Sullivan 1930), and the two men were at best passing acquaintances, the respective staffs saw themselves in deadly earnest competition. Thus when Gates heard of Rockefeller's idea to set up the educational fund along with Carnegie, he responded:

> "Mr. Carnegie's intimate friends tell me that it is no secret between them and him that he does these things for the sake of having his name written in stone all over the country. Have you observed that he always gives buildings while someone else furnishes the money to keep them in proper repair? Some of us cannot help thinking that these buildings are deemed by him as so many monuments to Andrew Carnegie, while others give the endowment funds to keep them up. ... Now this scheme of a central endowment fund is, I think, a most creditable one. But if you yoke up with Mr. Carnegie in it, he will somehow or other manage to absorb the whole thing and use your connection with it simply as the tail to his kite. I would like to let this plan come out as a great contrast to Mr. Carnegie's scheme, its wisdom, its efficiency, its promise of good for the community at large. You have the reputation, not only for giving, but for wise and skillful giving ... fair and thoughtful men will approve not alone

the gift but the giver of the gift. If you should make the proposition to the General Education Board, in a letter to be made public, and should point out how you wish this fund to be administered, Mr. Carnegie would have afforded him a clear example, which he could then follow. ... I have not much doubt that Mr. Carnegie would be willing to put in ten or twenty millions, but I should like for every reason just now to see you act, and act before Mr. Carnegie. It is not at all unlikely that if Mr. Carnegie gets the idea, he will immediately act on it, in advance of you, and secure the credit of it. Carnegie is putting his ten millions into a pension fund for teachers. I think this an act of extraordinary folly. Of all people teachers should be examples of thrift, of careful living within their means, and of hoarding up by small economies something against a rainy day. ... Mr. Carnegie is doing what he can, in this ten million dollar pension fund, to render thrift needless, superfluous and contemptible." [Gates Papers, Rockefeller Family Archives, April 24, 1905]

Gates kept up his written barrage against Carnegie until Rockefeller dropped the idea of working jointly:

"I do not share the fears of those who think the millionaire is a dangerous menace to the liberties of our people. The danger in him, I think, really is in a most expected quarter—that is—that he will relieve by lavish and unthinking benevolence the ordinary citizen from the need and reward of personal interest in, and contribution to, the general weal of the local community. Mr. Carnegie in his library schemes and more recently in his pension scheme is in my opinion a fit illustration of the millionaire as menace ..." [Gates Papers, Rockefeller Family Archives, May 24, 1905]

While Gates was not able to realize the ideal organization that he dreamed of, the GEB with its $10 million to be used solely for the creation of a system of higher education in the United States did in some respects come close. The Board accepted as its policy certain conditions that would ensure the type of educational system that he envisioned: money would be given for endowment only and not for operating expenses; money would be given only to institutions able to raise a certain amount on their own (matching grants, first pioneered by the Peabody Fund); the schools supported would be located in centers of wealth so that they could attract other local philanthropy; money would be given only to private (non-public) schools; the gifts would be contractual and hence conditions legally binding (Fosdick 1962).

4
Medicine in Chicago

In the study of philanthropic foundation involvement in medicine and medical care, three phases of involvement can be identified. While they cannot be dated with exact precision, the attempt to periodize them helps in understanding their influence. The first phase stems from the 1890s to the publication of the Flexner Report in 1910. In this period, foundations helped to develop the physical resources and infrastructure (laboratories, equipment, facilities, manpower) necessary for a system of scientific medicine and medical care. The second phase stems from the publication of the Flexner Report in 1910 through the mid-1930s, and is the period of foundation aid to medical education for the development of physicians trained in a scientific manner. The third phase begins in the mid-1930s and extends into the present. It is the period of foundation involvement with medical policy change with the ultimate purpose of shifting the locus of financial support onto government. This chapter will concentrate primarily on the first phase of philanthropic foundation involvement with scientific medicine.

A note must be made of the foundations to be studied. In the period 1890–1910 the only large foundations (i.e. with assets over $1 million) operating in the field of medicine were the Rockefeller philanthropies (including the Rockefeller General Education Board, Rockefeller Institute for Medical Research and the Rockefeller Sanitary Commission) and to some extent the

Carnegie Foundation. E.V. Hollis, in his seminal work *Philanthropic Foundations and Higher Education* (1939), noted that over 90 per cent of the foundation grants made to higher education in the period 1902-34 were made by just nine foundations. The Rockefeller philanthropies account for over 73 per cent of the total foundation money going to higher education and the Carnegie philanthropies account for another 22 per cent. Thus over 95 per cent of all foundation money going to benefit higher education in this period, can be accounted by just the Carnegie and Rockefeller philanthropies (Hollis 1939: 268). This dominance is reason enough to center the discussion on these two philanthropies alone. This book, therefore, will deal primarily with these two foundations.

It might be useful to outline at the outset the amount of money for which foundations were responsible in medicine. Of the total $340,996,400 of philanthropic foundation support to higher education between 1902 and 1934, Hollis estimates that over $154 million (45 per cent) went specifically to medicine and medical education excluding such related and allied areas as public health, psychiatry, and life sciences not in medical schools (1939: 217). Abraham Flexner estimated that when alumni contribution and local philanthropy were included with the foundation grants, the total amount of money that went to medical education was over $600 million(1952: 57)

The University of Chicago–Rush Medical College Affair

The first inklings of the Rockefeller philanthropic direction in the field of medical science came during discussions and arguments over the affiliation/merger of the Rush Medical College with the University of Chicago in 1894, 1898, and later on in the early 1900s. These discussions took place before the creation of the Rockefeller Institute and were, in many ways, instrumental in shaping the philanthropic policies in medicine for the Rockefellers and, by implication, for other philanthropies as well. The importance of this episode in the history of the Rockefeller philanthropies can be gleaned from the fact that the Chicago dealings directed later Rockefeller money away from the

Medicine in Chicago

academic setting so that control over activities could be assured and maintained. The central importance of Frederick T. Gates and the corollary lesser significance of John D. Rockefeller, Sr. to the Rockefeller philanthropies can also be observed.

The University of Chicago was Rockefeller's first large philanthropic project. Originally a small and failing Baptist institution in Chicago, it was built, primarily through Rockefeller's support, into one of the leading private universities in the world. In the 1880s the American Baptist Education Society, an organization composed of Baptist ministers interested in promoting Baptist education throughout the United States, decided it was time to build a great Baptist university. The society was split over the location of the proposed school, with some members wanting it located in New York and others wanting it located in Chicago. At that time, Chicago was the leading city of the mid-west and an area of growing industrial importance in the United States. The city, however was sorely lacking an educational facility of note.

The richest Baptist in the world at that time was Rockefeller, Sr., and naturally the ABES turned to him for financial support of their plan. The leaders had only the most abstract plans for their university and were undecided as to its location. This lack of specificity combined with the intense pressure placed on him, led Rockefeller to shy away from making a commitment to the venture (Goodspeed 1916; Nevins 1904:191–265; Storr 1966). Realizing the mistake that the ABES leaders were making, Gates, Corresponding Secretary of the Society, prepared a detailed plan for the development of such a university in Chicago. Meeting Rockefeller, Sr. on a railroad trip, Gates purposely avoided the subject, waiting for Rockefeller to raise it. Rockefeller was impressed with Gates's style as well as by the cogent and detailed nature of Gates's report on the university. He was won over and his original gift of $600,000 was soon followed by many others: Rockefeller's contributions to the University amounted to over $35 million by the late 1930s (Gates 1977:102–07; Storr 1966).

At the time, Chicago was the home to fifteen medical schools, all proprietary. Twenty years later, Flexner would call the city "the plague spot of the country in respect to medical education" (Flexner 1960:87).

Rush Medical College was founded in 1843, just six years after the city of Chicago was incorporated (Hirsch 1966: 74). As was the custom with American medical schools of the time, the faculty of the college were also its trustees. Rush was a proprietary medical school devoted to the regular (allopathic) sect of medicine, the predominant mode of medicine in America at the time. Its reputation was based in part on its vocal rejection of homeopathy and other medical sects. Its faculty in the 1890s comprised a distinguished list of physicians including Frank Billings, Arthur Dean Bevan, Nicholas Senn, Ludwig Hektoen, and Edwin Klebs.

Medical schools with pretensions toward academia attempted to form affiliations with colleges and universities. The affiliation would give academic legitimacy to the medical school faculty and give the school the illusion of an intellectual connection or bond with an academic enterprise. Colleges and universities saw in affiliations extensions of their domains and thus valued them as well. The Rush Medical College had had an affiliation with the older University of Chicago but with the demise of that institution, it had worked out an affiliation agreement with Lake Forest College. As soon as the new University of Chicago was founded in 1892, there were inquiries from Rush about an affiliation. On May 11, 1892 Dr. E. Fletcher Ingals, Dean of the Rush Medical College, wrote to William Rainey Harper, President of the University of Chicago informing him that Rush would be willing to break off its affiliation with Lake Forest and re-establish its prior affiliation with the University of Chicago (Presidential Papers, University of Chicago archives).

While nothing came of this at the time, Ingals kept in touch with Harper, even asking him on December 2, 1892 to try and help Rush secure $250,000 for medical research (Presidential Papers, University of Chicago archives). According to Richard Storr (1966: 142), Harper was receptive to these offers of affiliation with Rush for several reasons: 1) the school was well known throughout Chicago; 2) it had a distinguished faculty; and 3) it had access to clinical teaching material at the Presbyterian hospital. Although Rush was in debt, it was the most promising medical school in Chicago at the time. Harper had been discussing the situation with Ingals and even began working out a tentative affiliation agreement. On January 27, 1894, Ingals wrote Harper to say that he had modified the agreement to read: "The property and goodwill of Rush Medical College to be transferred to the University of Chicago on condition that it shall always be maintained as a broad scientific school of medicine, as this term shall be understood by the majority of educated physicians throughout the world"(Presidential Papers, University of Chicago Archives).

On January 31, 1894, the agreement having been worked out between the two schools, Harper contacted Rockefeller and Gates in New York. Although both were members of the Board of Trustees, Rockefeller did not attend the Trustee meetings, since it was widely understood that Gates represented Rockefeller on the Board. Given the magnitude of Rockefeller's gifts to the University and its hope for continued largesse, it was unlikely that the University would do anything without his approval being sought, and it was expected that he would be kept informed of all events occurring at the University. It is noticeable in this regard that the stationery of the University bore the inscription "founded by John D. Rockefeller" under the name University of Chicago. It should also be noted that Gates had a considerable interest in the school given the efforts he had made and the role he played in bringing the University of Chicago into existence.

Homeopathy and allopathy were the two major competing sects in American medicine at this time. While there were other forms of healing including botanical medicine, herbalism, Thompsonian medicine, and eclectic medicine, homeopathy and allopathy were the only two that demanded a professional education and a M.D. degree.

Homeopathy was based on the theory that the symptoms that a body exhibited during an illness were an expression of the body's own attempt at self-cure. The therapy associated with this medicine involved trying to increase or expand the symptoms that the body exhibited. Additionally, homeopathy held that only the most minuscule dosages of drugs were necessary to get the body to respond. It was an extremely minimalist medicine and its appeal was primarily to the very wealthy, the very poor, women, and children because it was very cheap, very delicate, and generally very safe. Allopathy was based on the belief that the purpose of

A System of Scientific Medicine

medicine was not to augment symptoms but rather to try to eliminate them. The therapy of allopathy consisted of extremely heavy doses of very potent chemicals and drugs and other treatments including bleeding and purging. The members of the two schools did not mix as they were in serious economic competition with one another (Berliner 1975).

It should be noted that Rockefeller was a homeopath, that is he believed in and used physicians and medications that were homeopathic (Nevins 1940: 263). When news of the proposed affiliation reached New York, Rockefeller was against the affiliation because Rush was not a homeopathic school and he did not want to support an allopathic school. He was perhaps concerned by the portion of the agreement quoted above referring to a scientific school of medicine as defined by the majority of physicians which might be interpreted as advocating allopathy, the majority sect at the time. Gates was also against the affiliation, preferring to build his own school and thus have more control over it. On March 5, 1894 Gates wrote to Thomas W. Goodspeed (Secretary of the University of Chicago) and Harper regarding the Rush Medical College, noting that he had conferred with Rockefeller and that:

> "Mr. Rockefeller regards the matter as of very serious import and thinks that no step should be taken without the most careful and exhaustive inquiry and mutual consent. ... In view of the gravity of the matter, Mr. Rockefeller would prefer not to form any conclusion at present but to hold the matter in solution. Sometime when you are in New York, and he can see you, he will consult with you on the subject." [Goodspeed Papers, University of Chicago Archives]

Gates revealed in a letter several years later reviewing the course of events (January 12, 1898) that:

> "It [the relationship with Rush] was brought up early in 1894 and was seriously discussed and referred to counsel here, with correspondence with Dr. Harper, we then taking the ground that the union would be illegal. Indeed, I found Mr. Rockefeller very reluctant to form any relationship at the time and he adopted his usual mild course in such cases of laying the matter on the table, rather than giving a direct 'No'." [Goodspeed Papers, University of Chicago Archives]

Medicine in Chicago

With Rockefeller and Gates so firmly against any action being taken, the matter was laid to rest, at least for the time being. Although there were occasional references to medical schools in the correspondence between Gates and Rockefeller in New York and Harper and Goodspeed in Chicago, little occurred until 1897. Many rumors passed between East and Mid-west prompting Rockefeller on one occasion (December 18, 1895) to write to Gates:

> "Memorandum for Mr. Gates: It has been intimated to me that there was something about an allopathic department of medicine at the University. If we are to have a department of medicine there, I am a strong homeopathist and would desire that in medicine as well as in all other departments we should be aggressive. J.D.R." [Goodspeed Papers, University of Chicago Archives]

Gates immediately forwarded this letter to Harper in Chicago. In response, Harper wrote back to Gates on December 20, 1895:

> "My own opinion is that the best plan is to have a medical school which is neither homeopathic nor allopathic but simply scientific; in other words make an entirely new departure and, as Mr. Rockefeller says, be aggressive." [Rockefeller Family Archives, Educational Interests]

Harper was being pressured by the faculty at Rush to do something with medicine in Chicago even if it meant setting up a new school. In his Presidential Convocation address of April 1, 1897 Harper devoted some attention to the subject:

> "What is the greatest single piece of work which still remains to be done for the cause of education in the city of Chicago and in connection with the University? ... A School of Medicine in the city of Chicago, with an endowment large enough to make it independent of the fees received from its students, with an endowment large enough to provide instruction of as high an order as any that may be found in European cities, with an endowment large enough to provide the facilities of investigation and research which may be used by those who would devote their time to the study of methods of prevention of disease as well as the cure of disease; an endowment for medicine which would make it unnecessary for men to seek lands beyond the sea for the sake of doing work which ought to be done here at home; such an endowment, I assert, for medical education,

A System of Scientific Medicine

is the greatest piece of work which still remains to be done for the cause of education in the city of Chicago. It is impossible to conceive the far-reaching results of such an act. Our children through all the generations would enjoy the benefits of such a benefaction. The poor throughout the crowded districts of our city would be more directly benefited in this way than in any other. Men of learning tell us that we are only *entering* upon the field of medical science. If this is true, what greater boon to humanity than a foundation which shall make possible more rapid progress, more extensive achievement? ... I do not have in mind an institution of charity, or an institution which shall devote itself merely to the the education of a man who shall be an ordinary physician; but rather an institution which shall occupy a place beside the two or three such institutions that already exist in our country, one whose aim shall be to push forward the boundaries of medical science, one in which honor and distinction will be found for those only who make contributions to the cause of medical science, one from which announcements may be sent from time to time so potent in their meaning as to stir the whole civilized world. There is no other work which will lift our beloved city of Chicago more quickly to a place of honor and esteem among the cities of the world. There is no other deed, the advantage of which would accrue more directly or more abundantly to this city of which we are so justly proud. I plead, men and women of Chicago, for a School of Medicine which shall be the equal to any which today exists; for such an institution which will draw from all parts of the world men and women who shall find incentive and opportunity to do something for the mitigation of human suffering, for the amelioration of human life." [Goodspeed 1916: 330–31]

Storr pointed out that this speech was remarkably similar in content to a letter that had been sent to Harper by Ingals, Dean of Rush Medical College, suggesting that he talk on this topic (1966:143). Harper was careful not to commit himself to very much, talking only of medical work to be done "in connection with the University". In December 1897, the University again listened to the pleas of Rush for a merger. The University agreed to an affiliation only if Rush would meet stringent conditions. These included: 1) Rush had to agree to replace its present trustees (i.e., its faculty) with a completely new set of outside trustees; faculty could have no pecuniary interest in the running of the school; 2) Rush had to pay off all its debts; 3) admission requirements were to be raised to a minimum of two years of college by 1902. Rush agreed to these terms hoping that adherence would lead to an eventual union or organic merger rather than just the affiliation that was being discussed (Storr 1966:144). Rush's interest lay primarily in the anticipated bequests that Rockefeller might be making in the near future.

The discussions between Rush and the University were kept quiet and occurred entirely in Chicago, perhaps due to the fear that the New York people would once again be negative toward affiliation. This in fact proved to be the case. The University officially let Gates know that it was seriously considering an affiliation with Rush on January 10, 1898. While Gates was disturbed that the matter had not been discussed with him previously, he was even more disturbed that the last time he had mentioned the matter to Harper, the President had played down the activity that clearly had been going on. In his response to Goodspeed on January 12, 1898 Gates said:

> "I was opposed to the affiliation when Dr. Harper was here and so indicated, in a general way, when he made a somewhat casual reference to it. I will not state the general grounds of my opposition, one being with me decisive and that is that Mr. Rockefeller has been and is opposed to allopathic medicine." [Goodspeed Papers, University of Chicago Archives]

Gates continued with a general history of the affiliation story to date and how he and Rockefeller had been opposed to the affiliation from the start and had thus assumed the matter to be at an end. Gates reiterated Rockefeller's stand in favor of homeopathy and against allopathy toward which Rockefeller felt that "we should be aggressive". Gates continued:

> "This was conclusive as to Mr. Rockefeller's desire that at least no relationship should be entered into with allopathic institutions. In addition to the above, the matter has frequently been talked over and it has been well understood what Mr. Rockefeller's views on these matters are. I have no doubt that Mr. Rockefeller would favor an institution that was neither allopath or homeopath but simply scientific in its investigation of medical science. That is the ideal. For that

A System of Scientific Medicine

the University should wait and reserve the great weight of its influence, authority and prestige instead of bestowing the same gratuitously on Rush Medical College. Such an institution would have to be endowed and would be run on a far higher principle than the principle of Rush College or any other of the ordinary institutions."

This paragraph was pregnant with intent and possibility. Here was Gates committing Rockefeller, albeit indirectly, to endowing a school of medicine. Yet it does not seem to follow from Rockefeller's own attitudes toward medicine. He had clearly stated that he wanted a homeopathic school and was against the merger because Rush was not homeopathic. Yet Gates implies that Rockefeller wanted as he did, a scientific school. In a letter sent to Goodspeed on December 28, 1915, Gates justified this position by saying:

"Mr. Rockefeller read this letter and this passage in the letter before it was sent. He read this quasi-committal of himself to such an institution for Chicago had the way been left open for it, and he allowed it to be sent by his official representative. There can be therefore, no doubt at all that Mr. Rockefeller did cherish the ideals and plans which you attribute to him and one of his objections at least against the affiliation of Rush was that Rush Medical College did not offer a suitable foundation for the ideal which he had in mind, an ideal which ultimately was realized in the Rockefeller Institute for Medical Research." [Rockefeller Family Archives, Educational Interests]

In another reminiscence of these events, this to Starr J. Murphy on December 31, 1915 Gates wrote:

"In the original letter, and in my letterbook copy from which I take this quotation, these words were made the central point of the entire letter by running along the margin of each side a heavy line [the words about the institution being neither homeopathic nor allopathic]. ... My purpose was to intimate to Dr. Goodspeed, official secretary of the University, to whom the letter was addressed, that this passage contained for him a pregnant meaning. I intended to intimate to him that if he would quietly wait, the founder would probably endow an institute of research in connection with the University of Chicago. Mr. Rockefeller understood the implication of these words of course as well as I did, and he not only permitted, but ordered the letter to be sent with all the implications that it contained." [Corner 1965:582]

It is not clear that Rockefeller actually did feel the way Gates described. His own statements showed that he did not favor a scientific school but very clearly wanted a homeopathic one. Rockefeller continued to support homeopathy against scientific medicine for quite some time despite numerous and important benefactions made in his name to scientific medicine. For example, in a letter to Dr. Harper written on June 30, 1905, Rockefeller encouraged Harper to seek osteopathic treatment for an ailment that Harper was suffering: "The name of the osteopathist who gave me treatment is Dr. J. G. Helmer, No. 136 Madison Avenue, and I am satisfied I have received no little benefit from this treatment. I have steadily improved" (Presidential Papers, University of Chicago Archives). One can only conclude that it was Gates who favored the scientific approach and not Rockefeller.

It was at this time that Gates began to get involved in a study of scientific medicine and had even written to Harper during the summer of 1897 to tell him of his interest in reading Osler's *Textbook of Medicine* (Rockefeller Family Archives, Gates Philanthropy).

To return to the Gates-Harper/Goodspeed correspondence, Gates continued his letter of January 12, 1898 by saying that he was against either a merger or an affiliation. He concluded by saying:

> "I believe that the vote of the board, affiliating Rush Medical College, was a very serious blunder in the development of the University of Chicago. This is not from Mr. Rockefeller's point of view alone, but from the point of view of the best development of the institution, quite apart from Mr. Rockefeller's personal views respecting schools of medicine, although in saying this I am not to be understood as relieving the emphasis of his personal wishes in the matter."

Goodspeed responded on January 15, 1898 most apologetically, stating that Dr. Harper had not tried to deceive Gates. The question of a merger had been turned down but the Board agreed to a loose affiliation. Goodspeed wrote:

> "After his [Harper's] return [from a New York meeting with Gates]

simple affiliation was proposed by Dr. Ingals such as we have entered into with Colleges and Academies. This was a wholly new proposal in strict accordance with the policy of the University which we had understood to be approved and warmly approved from the very inception of the enterprise. I do not think it occurred to the Trustees that the School of Medicine to which Rush belonged was a matter of interest or weight where the question was merely one of affiliation. When the question was asked in our board meeting 'What good will this do to the University', Mr. Ryerson [Chairman of the Board] answered, 'That is not the question. The University is here to uplift education in the West and the question is, "Shall we in this, advance the cause of medical education".' [Rockefeller Family Archives, Educational Interests]

Goodspeed reiterated the point about the school of medicine being unimportant:

"Thus the question of the School of Medicine to which Rush belonged was not thought to be important when a simple affiliation was desired. It belonged to a reputable school and that was enough. The affiliation had not committed the University in the slightest degree to allopathy. If a homeopathic school in Chicago with the high standing of Rush should apply for affiliation we could have no reason for refusing it. ... I understand it to be the policy of the University not to take part in the controversy between the Schools of Medicine, but to encourage both the great Schools. When the University has a medical department of its own, it will fill it with professors of both schools. In this respect the views of our trustees agree perfectly with those of Mr. Rockefeller, of whom you say 'I have no doubt that he would favor an institution that was neither allopath or homeopath but simply scientific in its investigation of medical science. That is the ideal.' To this we assent cordially, warmly, unanimously. For this we wait and hope and pray."

Goodspeed concluded the letter by saying that "the Trustees would not on any consideration go counter to Mr. Rockefeller's wishes."

In retrospect, it seems that Goodspeed misinterpreted the dynamics of the Rockefeller organization. By writing to appease what he presumed was Rockefeller's unhappiness with the situation (merger or affiliation with an allopathic rather than a homeopathic school), he made relations worse with Gates. The last thing that Gates wanted to hear was that the University would give equal time to homeopathy. Gates was interested in scientific medicine only and the idea that the University still thought in terms of sects infuriated Gates. Moreover, Gates was not swayed by the sophistry of Goodspeed's letter. He wrote in the margin of his copy of the letter that the question that Harper and he had discussed was affiliation and not merger as Goodspeed had suggested.

Gates responded on January 19, 1898 in a letter addressed to both Harper and Goodspeed. He starts by getting the issue of homeopathy out of the way:

"I regret it all the more because Dr. Harper, no less than myself, does not agree with Mr. Rockefeller's views regarding homeopathy, and we would both look with some concern as to the direction with which the medical department of the University might take. These are unfortunate coincidences for all of these considerations pointed with the utmost possible emphasis to a frank discussion of the whole matter with Mr. Rockefeller before any action was taken. I regret the kind of action that was taken of posing heavy burdens on the college and leaving what the University should do nearly a blank sheet of paper to be filled in afterwards." [Goodspeed Papers, University of Chicago Archives]

Gates continued:

"The effect of the matter will be that any one desiring to endow medical education in Chicago, even if nothing further is said, will feel that the tremendous force of the University of Chicago is brought to bear upon them to put their endowments into Rush. This is the very purpose of the whole thing with Rush at least. The whole effect and tendency of this movement will be to make Rush ultimately the medical department of the University of Chicago as against that far higher and better conception, *which has been one of the dreams of my own mind at least*, of a medical college in this country conducted by the University of Chicago, magnificently endowed, devoted primarily to investigation, making practice itself an incident of investigation and taking as its students only the choicest spirits, quite irrespective of the question of funds. Against this ideal and possibility a tremendous, if not fatal, current has been turned. I believed the ideal to be quite practicable and I hoped to live to see it realized. The University, however, has in this action, to all intents and purposes in the public mind, turned over the whole thing to Rush Medical College." [emphasis added]

Apparently, as he was writing this letter, the *University Record* for January 14, 1898 crossed his desk. This issue announced the Rush affiliation to the University of Chicago community. In the article on the affiliation, Harper praised Rush Medical College and talked about the future of the affiliation:

"This proposition, which has already been adopted by the present trustees of Rush Medical College, is a most significant step in the history of medical education. ... It will be the aim of the new Trustees [of Rush], with such assistance as the University may furnish, to develop the work of the Medical College along University lines. ... Whether Rush Medical College will ever become the Medical College of the University, time will show. It is important, however, to note that even with this affiliation of Rush Medical College, the University remains without a medical school of its own. The field is therefore open for some friend of humanity to devote one or two millions of dollars for the endowment of a great medical school, the income of which shall be devoted to special research, with which under any circumstances Rush Medical College would work in the the closest cooperation ... " [University of Chicago 1898: 322]

Gates was further infuriated by these comments. In a postscript to his letter of January 19, 1898 he added:

"I do not need to comment on this language. It simply justifies everything I have said. It is nothing to the point that Dr. Harper says other things of a qualifying nature in this address. He does, indeed, make a halfhearted and perfunctory suggestion that somebody should give some two millions to endow the university a medical department of its own, qualifying the very suggestion with the words '*even* with this affiliation, etc., the University remains without a medical school of its own,' although the sentence immediately preceding states it is an open question whether Rush Medical College will not be such a school. What Dr. Harper says looking toward ultimate union will be sounded out, from one end of Chicago to the other and as far as the alumni of Rush are scattered, with the voice of Gabriel's trumpet, awaking the dead, while his qualifying phrases will not have the voice of a pewee."

Harper still thought the problem lay with Rockefeller, Sr.'s aversion to allopathy and that Gates was just orating and rhetorically relating his employer's feelings. He corresponded with Dean Ingals of Rush on the subject and the Dean came up with a letter for Harper to send to New York which he assumed would square things. On January 24, 1898 Ingals wrote to Harper:

"I enclose a letter which may be of service to you in dealing with our friends in New York. I have in it stated as clearly as possible our position in this matter and it seems to me that reasonable men whatever their beliefs about medicine, should be able to comprehend it." [Presidential Papers, University of Chicago Archives]

The friends in New York were a reference to Gates and Rockefeller. Ingals's plan was to teach medical students homeopathy in such a way that they would themselves reject it as a useless doctrine. This way, they satisfied both the need to include homeopathy for Rockefeller's sake and their own interest in disposing of it. The letter, which was to be shown to the people in New York, was from Ingals to Harper and dated January 24, 1898:

"Regarding homeopathy, my colleagues and I believe that medical students should be taught all that is known of medical science. In the subjects of Anatomy, Physiology, Chemistry, Obstetrics, Surgery, Pathology and the Diagnosis of disease, there can be no possible difference of opinion between the educated homeopathist and the educated regular physician. Therefore all differences are confined to the subject of Materia Medica and Therapeutics. If in homeopathy there are truths in this subject, they should be taught to all students. If this subject, as taught by homeopathy, will not bear investigation, there is no way so sure of demonstrating the error as to teach it thoroughly to students who are thoroughly educated in medical science. We believe therefore that it would be a good plan to have the subject taught in our regular schools." [Presidential Papers, University of Chicago Archives]

Furthermore, Harper was still under the impression that the issue was the sectarian identity of the affiliated institution. In a letter written to Martin Ryerson, Chairman of the Board of

Trustees of the University of Chicago, on March 24, 1898 Harper wrote:

> "Care was taken in the statements concerning Rush Medical College to state that no union would be effected until the conditions were complied with. Our friends in New York have been quite a little troubled with this matter, but I think that everything will be straightened out in due time. The real trouble, of course, is that Mr. Rockefeller is a homeopath and is somewhat disturbed concerning the allopathic tendency indicated in the proposed alliance." [Harper Papers, University of Chicago Archives]

Harper, Goodspeed and the Trustees all apologized to Gates and Rockefeller for not having consulted with them about the affiliation. As far as Gates was concerned, the damage was already done. After completing the requirements set out for it in the affiliation agreement in 1902, and after some additional fights, Rush became for a time the medical school of the University of Chicago. Gates would never have anything favorable to say about medicine in Chicago. The University had lost the chance to become the research institute that had been implied in Gates's letter—a school where teaching would be incidental to research and which would ignore, for all intents and purposes, the needs of the ordinary practitioner of medicine. It is of course not at all clear that anyone in Chicago wanted a school that matched Gates's vision. The Trustees of the University certainly did not share his view and the Rush faculty did not either (Hirsch 1966:103–04). While they considered research important, they saw the primary purpose of medical education as training doctors who would be in community practice.

In August 1902, Rockefeller was considering giving money to Rush Medical College. Gates dissuaded him from this, saying in a letter that he had already endowed the Rockefeller Institute for Medical Research (1901) and there was no need to waste money on Rush. If the Institute wanted to give grants to researchers at Rush, that was appropriate, however that should be the only money Rush should get (Rockefeller Family archives, Educational Interests, August 8, 1902).

As an interesting postscript to this story, it seems that Gates felt particularly guilty about discouraging his employer from supporting Rush. The same day that he wrote the above cited note in which he railed against giving any money to Rush, he started to write a letter to Goodspeed (August 8, 1902) which he apparently decided not to send. The letter began, "If you are good natured this morning, and I never knew you otherwise, read this letter. If you are not in the best of good nature, postpone it until sometime when you feel equal to taking a joke." Gates continues by giving a resumé of the entire Rush affair, pointing out his opposition to the affiliation from the beginning. He continued:

> "How little any of us can plan for the future. Since the days of the affiliation of Rush and the earnest correspondence between New York and Chicago thereon, what changes have taken place! Changes in Rush and perhaps in the University which make it seem desirable and feasible to the Board of Trustees, who then repudiated such a thought, that Rush be incorporated into the University as the foundation of its medical department. This I foresaw. But I did not imagine at that time that Mr. Rockefeller could or would be led to the establishment of the Rockefeller Institute of [sic] Medical Research, that within two years he would have paid $1,200,000 into it, for work of research, that he would not only dissociate it from Rush Medical Center but from any medical college ... but that he would go further and would dissociate it wholly from the University of Chicago and from the City of Chicago, and establish it as an independent institution conducted by the best medical experts of the entire country and located solely with reference to the best possible work." [Rockefeller Family Archives, Educational Interests]

As the next chapter will show, the lesson that Gates learned from his Chicago experience was that a university was not necessarily the best organizational solution to a problem, especially if it were geographically distant and maintained its independence. Gates would not again make the mistake of leaving important decisions to the administrators of a university. He would, instead, make the decisions himself and give the institution a take-it-or-leave-it choice.

The problems of the affiliation between the University of Chicago and Rush apparently led Gates into serious consideration of scientific medicine for the first time. Thereafter it is

A System of Scientific Medicine

apparent that while the money was supplied by Rockefeller, the policies were made by Gates. As time went on, Gates took an increasingly more active and open role in making policy within the Rockefeller philanthropies.

5
The Establishment of the Rockefeller Institute

Although originally named the Rockefeller Institute for Medical Research, and now called Rockefeller University, the first major medical research institution in the United States was actually conceived not by a member of the Rockefeller family but by Gates. Rockefeller, Jr., who also played a key role in the founding of the Institute attested to Gates's contribution in a memorial speech to Gates upon his death in 1929. Rockefeller, Jr. said: "... for the institute was conceived in his own mind; it was the child of his own brain"(1929:2).

Most histories of medical research and philanthropy describe how Gates got the idea for an institution devoted to scientific medical research after reading William Osler's *Principles and Practice of Medicine* during the summer of 1897. There are however three different interpretations of what led Gates to read this book in the first place. They are attributed to: 1) the initial attempt of the University of Chicago-Rush Medical College affiliation in 1894; 2) a personal illness Gates had; 3) his perceptions of the deficiencies of medicine based on his early pastorate experience.

When the University of Chicago first proposed an affiliation with the Rush Medical College in 1894, Gates opposed the merger for reasons never made specific but presumably because Rockefeller, Sr. did not want to support an allopathic school. It seems likely that Gates's interest in medicine was piqued by the battles over the affiliation. As noted in the last chapter, it was to

A System of Scientific Medicine

President Harper of Chicago that Gates wrote to tell of reading Osler's book.

Simon Flexner, in the eulogy for Gates, said:

"The project of an institution for medical research ... originated in Mr. Gates' mind, grew out of his personal experience. Mr. Gates has told me about this. He had a very dangerous illness when he was in the prime of life. Escaping with his life, he decided to acquaint himself with the state of medical knowledge existing at the time." [1929:14]

Gates himself noted that it was his experiences in his early days in the pastorate in Minnesota that led him to question the effectiveness of the medicine of any school and search for an alternative:

"In the latter half [1884-88] of my pastorate in Minneapolis, there were in my congregation several practicing physicians, as well as the usual quota of faith healers, Christian Scientists and medical nondescripts, each not unwilling to have an encouraging word here and there from the pastor. ... To me the inference was obvious and inevitable that neither school was having much effect on the health of the community, and that even if there had existed a science of medicine, that science was not being taught or practiced in the United States. ... And so when I entered Mr. Rockefeller's private office in 1893 [*sic* 1891], I had been for years convinced that medicine as generally taught and practiced in the United States was practically futile. But I determined at length that I would find out what really lay in the minds of doctors in active practice. I would read the textbooks they studied." [1977:179-81]

For any one of these reasons or a combination of all three, Gates was led to read William Osler's textbook on medicine in the summer of 1897. Gates had spent the spring and early summer with a medical student at the College of Physicians and Surgeons, which was at that time loosely connected with Columbia University. The student was Elon O. Huntington whom he had known as a young boy. As Huntington was alone in New York he spent occasional weekends at the Gates home in Montclair, New Jersey during which he and Gates went for long walks and talks. Gates related much of their relationship and his introduction to medical literature in his autobiography:

"Thus, in simply entertaining Elon I found myself intensely interested in medicine. My interest reached a point in which I determined to know something more definite about medicine. ... In the spring of 1897 ... I told him [Elon] that I would like to read medicine, and I asked him if he could suggest to me a book which a layman like me might be able to understand and to read with profit. I remember telling him that I did not want any of the ordinary medical books for the family. I wanted to know what the best doctors are reading; I wanted the literature that was being taught currently in the best schools to medical students. Was there any such book preeminently good? He replied that there was one such book; it was Osler's *Principles and Practice of Medicine* ..." [Corner 1965: 575–84]

Gates purchased the book at a New York bookstore. The book had first appeared in 1892, and it appears that Gates read the second edition which was published in 1896 (1965: 23). Gates went on vacation during the summer of 1897 and took the book and a medical dictionary to the Catskill Mountains in New York with him.

"I read the whole book without skipping any of it. I speak of this not to commemorate my industry but to illustrate Osler's charm. ... There was a fascination about the style itself that led me on and having once started I found a hook in my nose that pulled me from page to page, and chapter to chapter, until the whole of about a thousand closely printed pages brought me to the end." [Corner 1965: 578]

Gates was impressed not only with the style of the book, but with its contents as well. He commented on the book in a letter he wrote to President Harper on June 19, 1897 concerning Harper's illness:

"You ought also to secure the very best diagnosis of your case. I think you ought to submit to a very close and critical examination from one or more eminent physicians covering the whole physical situation and learn from them accurately what organs, if any, are affected and the nature of your trouble. I am just now reading the recent book on the practice of medicine by the head of the Johns Hopkins Medical School [sic] and have scarcely ever read anything more intensely interesting." [Rockefeller Family Archives, Gates philanthropy]

In his autobiographical writings, Gates described his impressions of Osler's book. It should be noted that Gates produced many versions of his impressions of the book and the circumstances under which he read it and the outcome resulting from what he read. The first of these recollections was in 1915 and they continued through his autobiographical writings of 1926–28. The following is from his letter to Goodspeed :

> "I had been a sceptic before, not only as to homeopathic medicine but as to allopathic medicine as currently practiced. This book not only confirmed my scepticism, but its revelation absolutely astounded and appalled me, sceptic as I was. . . . I found, for illustration, that the best medical practice did not, and did not pretend to cure more than four or five diseases. That is medicine had, at that time, specifics for as many diseases as there are fingers on one hand. It was nature, and not the doctor, and in most instances nature practically unassisted, that performed the cures. I learned that with the exception of two or three, the physician had nothing whatever to prescribe for the infectious diseases, which could effect a cure. . . . To the layman student, like me, demanding cures, and specifics, he has no word of comfort whatever. In fact, I saw clearly from the work of this able and honest man, that medicine had, with few exceptions above mentioned, no cures, and that about all that medicine up to 1897 could do was to nurse the patients and alleviate in some degree the suffering. Beyond this, medicine as a science had not progressed. I found further that a large number of the most common diseases, especially of the young and middle aged, were simply infectious or contagious, were caused by infinitesimal germs that are breathed in with the atmosphere, or are imparted by contact or are taken in with the food or communicated by the incision of insects in the skin, which serves as a protective covering. I learned that of these germs, only a very few had been identified and isolated. I made a list, and it was a very long one at that time, much longer than it is now [1915], of the germs which we might reasonably hope to discover but which as yet had never been, with certainty, identified, and I made a very much longer list of the infectious or contagious diseases for which there had been as yet no specific found. When I laid down this book, I had begun to realize how woefully neglected in all civilized countries and perhaps most of all, in this country, had been the scientific study of medicine. I saw very clearly also why this was true. In the first place, the instruments of investigation, the microscope, the science of chemistry, had not until recently been developed. Pasteur's

Establishment of the Rockefeller Institute

germ theory of disease was very recent. Moreover while other departments of science, astronomy, chemistry, physics, etc., had been endowed very generously in colleges and universities throughout the whole civilized world, medicine, owing to the peculiar commercial organization of medical colleges, had rarely, if ever, been anywhere endowed, and research and instruction alike had been left to shift for itself dependent altogether on such chance as the active practitioner might steal from his practice. It became clear to me that medicine could hardly hope to become a science until medicine should be endowed and qualified men could give themselves to uninterrupted study and investigation, on ample salary, entirely independent of practice. To this end, it seemed to me that an Institute of medical research ought to be established in the United States. Here was an opportunity, to me the greatest, which the world could afford, for Mr. Rockefeller to become a pioneer." [Corner 1965: 579-80]

Upon his return from vacation (autobiography and letter to Murphy say July 24, 1897; letter to Goodspeed August 24, 1897), Gates set out to do something about his vision. Below is Gates's own description of the letter he wrote to Rockefeller. Since this letter has been lost, only Gates's recollection of it remains:

"I enumerated the infectious diseases and pointed out how few of the germs had yet been discovered and how great the field of discovery, how few specifics had yet been found and how appalling was the unremedied suffering. I pointed to the Koch Institute in Berlin and at greater length to the Pasteur Institute in Paris. It was either in this connection or a little later, for I kept up my inquiries on the subject, that I pointed out, as I remember the fact, that the results in dollars or francs of Pasteur's discoveries about anthrax and on the diseases of fermentation has saved for the French nation a sum far in excess of the entire cost of the Franco-German war. I remember insisting in this or some subsequent memorandum, that even if the proposed institute should fail to discover anything, the mere fact that he, Mr. Rockefeller, had established such an institute of research, if he were to consent to do so, would result in other institutes of a similar kind, or at least other funds for research being established, until research in this country would be conducted on a great scale and that out of the multitudes of workers, we might be sure in the end of abundant rewards even though those rewards did not come directly from the institute which he might found." [Corner 1965: 580]

Nevins commented on the Pasteur statement: "In writing this Gates was probably thinking of Huxley's famous statement that it had saved more than the indemnity paid by France" (1940: 469).

According to Gates, Rockefeller was on a business trip to Cleveland when this memo was drafted and Gates soon left for a long business trip to the Pacific coast. While there are no firm dates that can be verified, these events apparently took place in the fall of 1897. Thus Gates's firm position on the affiliation of Rush Medical College with the University of Chicago was influenced by his new-found understanding of the need for research. Gates's comments on his role in communicating Rockefeller's interests in a research institute demonstrate not only the confidence and power entrusted to him but his growing commitment to a system of scientific medicine. In a later explanation of his position toward the proposed merger, he explained:

> "You will observe here that the central thought is an institution for investigation. An institution in which whatever practice of medicine there is, shall be in itself an incident of investigation, that while I said this was a dream of my own I qualified by saying 'at least of my own mind' implying that it might also be a dream in another mind, and I not only stated that I believed it to be practical, but I added that I thought it was possible. This letter with all these implications, passed under the very critical eye of Mr. Rockefeller. He understood the implications perfectly, he knew perfectly well that those who read the letter, although I signed it, would understand and give just the same significance to it as if he signed it himself. I was acting as his secretary, if not his amanuensis in sending it. This statement, therefore, ... reveals still more clearly that the idea of a research institute had taken such possession of Mr. Rockefeller's mind that he was prepared to endorse the quasi public commitment to it which is made in his letter. But from this time forward, Mr. Rockefeller never associated the proposed institute with the University of Chicago." [Corner 1965: 583]

While Gates may have felt that this exonerated him from any blame in not giving a research institute to the University of Chicago, it in no way proves that Rockefeller, Sr. endorsed the idea of an institute devoted to scientific medicine. What little evidence there is suggests that Rockefeller had absolutely no idea

Establishment of the Rockefeller Institute

what scientific medicine was nor did he care. He remained committed to homeopathy, with brief excursions into osteopathic treatment, and avoided even visiting the Rockefeller Institute, once it was established.

While Rockefeller, Sr. may have had little to do with the policy directions and decision making that was going on in his name, his son, John D. Rockefeller, Jr., was just beginning to assume an active role in his father's philanthropic ventures. Having graduated from college, Rockefeller, Jr. came into the Rockefeller offices at 26 Broadway in 1897. He was given the choice of helping to accumulate the surplus or to distribute it. He chose the latter. As Nevins, in his biography of the elder Rockefeller put it:

> "Early in October [1897] he reported to 26 Broadway. His father did nothing either to push or guide the novice. 'He never said one word to me about what I was to do, nor did he say a word to anyone else in the office,' writes the son. 'He intended that I should make my own way.' By this time Rockefeller was withdrawing from the direction of the Standard [Oil Company] and seldom came downtown. The son had no difficulty in deciding that his career was to lie in dealing with the now colossal and constantly growing fortune—that is, in the work of investment and giving. If he had wished to be a money-maker he would have joined the management of the Standard as [uncle] William Rockefeller's oldest son did. But he was anxious to help protect the accumulations that already promised to become an ever-mounting burden, and distribute them for the public good. . . . Instead of going into Archibald's office [Director of Standard Oil], he entered that of Gates." [1940: 287]

It was soon after Gates and the younger Rockefeller teamed up that progress on the idea of a medical research institute began. Gates realized that before any prolonged and serious discussion could begin, an extensive study of existing research institutions would be necessary, as well as a conference with the leading medical men in Europe and America. Gates suggested that a friend and neighbor of his, Starr J. Murphy, be hired to "do whatever correspondence, and travel might be necessary in interviewing the leading men in the United States most intelligent on such a subject, and doing what reading might be necessary to inform himself more generally" (Corner 1965: 583). Rockefeller, Jr. met with Murphy, a lawyer by training, and approved of him, thereby allowing him to start work on this matter.

Tentative inquiries were made through Harvard University and Columbia University about a research institute on behalf of the Rockefeller family. President Seth Low of Columbia wrote to distinguished leaders in medical research in the United States and Britain including William H. Welch (Johns Hopkins), T. Mitchell Prudden (Bellevue), and Sir George Nuttall (Cambridge) in August, 1900 asking the following:

> "I am interested to ask you the following questions: [1] Would it be a matter of great advantage to medical science, and through it to humanity, if an institute on the same general lines as the Pasteur Institute in Paris were to be established in America and properly endowed? [2] If such an institute were to be established in the United States, where should it be located? That is to say, in what place would it be likely to accomplish the most good and most completely justify its foundation? [3] Should such an institute, in order to accomplish the most good, be a separate foundation, or should it be affiliated with a hospital or with a medical school? [4] What sort of results might be reasonably expected to follow the foundation of such an institute, properly endowed and equipped? [5] What do you think should be the working force of such an establishment and what endowment would it require in order to be as useful as possible? I shall be greatly obliged if, in replying to these questions, you will give briefly the reasons in each case upon which your opinions are based. I may add that this is not an idle inquiry, although I cannot say, on the other hand, that it will certainly lead to anything. The questions, however, deserve your most careful consideration. There is no immediate hurry for a reply." [Prudden 1927: 280–81]

Upon receiving answers from the three men, Low prepared a summary of their answers and sent them to Rockefeller, Jr. The summary that Low prepared is as follows:

> "1. The value of such an institution: Dr. Prudden: 'The advancement of medical science and the benefit to humanity which the founding and adequate endowment of such an institution in this country would secure can, in my opinion, hardly be overrated. I do not know of any other means by which with so much certainty individual suffering and misery could be relieved and prevented and research

fostered along lines involving the highest general welfare.' Dr. Nuttall: 'I can think of no way in which a wish to be truly philanthropic can be better realized and certainly a great country like the United States needs such an institution.' Dr. Welch: 'I am confident that the establishment in this country of a properly endowed institute on the general lines of the French Pasteur Institute be the greatest benefit to medical science and humanity. I know of no other way in which the expenditure of a like sum of money could be expected to yield greater results in the advancement of universal knowledge and in the physical well being of mankind.'

"2. The desirability of connecting with some university of standing: The advantages of such a connection are as follows: (1) Administration would be better for such a university could command a better quality of administrative ability than a separate institution could. (2) Such a connection would lend authority to the results of investigations. (3) The association of a community of interest would be of great help and stimulus. (4) It would make it easier to get the best quality of men as they value such university connections and many of them cannot connect themselves with such an institution without such university connection. (5) Cooperation of the various departments of the university would be valuable and through the medical departments especially, we could get access to hospitals.

"3. Plan and scope: The scope for research should not be limited by restrictions because it is at times impossible to tell the direction which an investigation will take or to foretell what may result from work which at the outset may appear to be irrelevant. It should cover the whole field of hygiene and preventive medicine. This should be somewhat broader in scope than the Pasteur Institute. The special conditions in this country strongly urge this variation in conception. The work should be divided into departments as no one man could possibly grasp more than a small part of what is required. The departments suggested — general hygiene, bacteriology-medical, bacteriology-industrial, parasitology, epidemiology—for the study of all the facts concerned in the origin and spread of epidemic and other infectious diseases, pathology-human, pathology-comparative, physiology, physics — for studies requiring accurate instrumental records including meteorology, chemistry-inorganic, chemistry-organic, especially the chemistry of life. If possible it would be well also to have departments of sanitary engineering and architecture and sanitary law and administration. The institute should have a large building or buildings for its various departments and also have a small tract of land outside the city for the care of experimental animals. If possible rooms should be provided in the building for a public museum of hygiene and sanitation. Large public lecture rooms with facilities for demonstrations; smaller lecture rooms and laboratories for investigation and advanced students and suites for working force. There should also be a library with provisions for records and statistical data. The provision should also be made for a publication fund and for special public lectures.

"4. Organization: There should be a council of men of science and medicine to make appointments. The heads of departments should be members of the council. The business affairs should be in the hands of the manager and assistants who should be men of business training but preferably university educated as well. The working force should consist of a director, head of departments, assistants in each department, fellows holding research fellowships granted for special merit, special students limited to those who have demonstrated special qualifications. There should be no teaching of undergraduates but it might be well to have the heads of the departments and associates and assistants each give a three month course during the year to advanced students in order to keep them from getting narrow in their views. There will also be needed a librarian and recorder to assist the workers and the researchers. Mechanic and general superintendent of plant, stenographers, attendants, etc. An appropriate degree might be given. The appointments should be entirely free from local considerations and should be open to the entire world. Where cooperation of departments is needed for special research they should be arranged for by the director. Each head of department should be left as free as possible.

"5. Endowment: Dr. Prudden thinks there should be an endowment of $100,000 a year. Dr. Welch thinks that if the best results were obtained the endowment should be $75,000 a year, Dr. Nuttall does not give any summary but suggests the following summaries—Chief of departments, $2,000–5,000; assistants, $1,000–1,500; research fellowships, $300–600. Chiefs and assistants to have every fifth year a leave of absence with full pay for travelling and observation abroad. The laboratories of the Royal College of Physicians and Surgeons in London have buildings costing 30,000 pounds and an annual expenditure of 1,500 pounds. The Jenner Institute of Preventive Medicine in London has buildings costing around 20,000 pounds and has recently received an endowment from Lord Iveagh of 250,000 pounds.

"6. Location: It should be located in or near a great city. Dr. Prudden does not express a preference, Dr. Welch prefers New York City because of its population and its importance as a port, its hospitals, libraries, medical schools, universities and its relation to the commercial and other interests of the rest of the country. Dr. Nuttall prefers Washington because of the unique library of the Surgeon-General's Office located in that city and considers the value of this will outweigh that of hospital facilities in New York. (Note: it seems to me that the benefits can be secured without locating the institute in Washington. It would be possible to have a special investigator located in Washington, with a suitable quota of assistants and stenographers who could make investigations in the libraries in Washington upon requisition for the workers in New York and abstract all necessary material and these abstracts could be placed on file in New York and would eventually become extremely valuable.)

"7. Results to be anticipated or attempted: — discovery of the specific germs of infectious diseases whose agents are not known, such as yellow fever, scarlet fever, etc.—larger knowledge of the properties and modes of distribution of known disease producing agents such as those of typhoid fever, tuberculosis, diptheria.—improved methods of diagnosis and prevention.—prevention and cure of mental disorder. — causation and cure of cancer and other malignant tumors.—preventative and curative methods of treatment.—improved methods of disinfection of rooms and clothing.—diffusion of knowledge with regard to public and personal hygiene and sanitation. Dr. Prudden makes the following statement: 'Four fifths of the existing suffering from disease and its attendant discomfort and misery are avoidable through the diffusion and application among the people of the knowledge of disease and its causes, which science has recently brought to light and which is now largely ignored.' Such an institution would also be a source of authoritative opinion with regard to the questions of the class covered by its investigations. Dr. Nuttall also suggests as fields of work the preparation and standardization of sera, bacteriological diagnosis—diptheria, etc., examination of water, sewerage, foods, etc. These, however, are already largely covered by the work done in this country by the city, state and federal authorities. It appears from the statements made by the representatives of the Harvard Medical School that it is arranging to fit men for work in medical laboratories. The establishment of such an institute as we contemplate would undoubtedly lead to the establishment of similar schools in all leading medical schools of the country which would furnish us with candidates and students for research fellowships." [Rockefeller Family Archives, Educational Interests, November 7, 1900]

Seth Low sent this summary to Rockefeller, Jr. on November 7, 1900. He also enclosed the following message:

"I have now the pleasure of handing you the two letters which I have received in response to a letter written by me from Northeast Harbor last summer, in regard to the matter about which you spoke to me last spring. In order that you may understand the significance of the replies, I send you a copy of the letter which has drawn them forth. Dr. Welch and Dr. Prudden would be universally considered, I think, two of the best authorities in the country upon this general subject. I have had no communication with either of them except that which is now submitted to you. I am interested to perceive that both of them think that such an institution in America would be likely to be most useful in connection with a university. Perhaps you will allow me to add to the reasons given by them this further consideration. That in the United States the best men value highly the university connection. If you wish any further service at my hands in this connection, please command me. Very truly yours, Seth Low."

This was the first contact that the Rockefeller people had with William H. Welch, a connection that was to become considerably more important over time, as Welch became the primary consultant on medical matters for the Rockefellers.

Although Rockefeller, Jr. was delivered into the world by a homeopathic physician, his own children were delivered and cared for by scientific physicians (Rockefeller Family Archives, Educational Interests, February 17, 1921). The pediatrician for his household was Dr. L. Emmett Holt, a renowned New York physician who attended the Fifth Avenue Baptist Church, as did the Rockefellers. Holt also took care of the children of Mrs. Harold Rockefeller McCormick of Chicago, Rockefeller, Jr.'s sister. Sometime during November, 1900, while Holt was returning from ministering to the McCormick children in Chicago, and Rockefeller, Jr. was returning from family business in Cleveland, the two met on a train from Cleveland to New York (Nevins 1940: 471). According to Holt, the following conversation took place:

"At that time the results of the application of diptheria antitoxin were still new and most impressive. I narrated to Mr. Rockefeller in considerable detail the steps of patient investigation and research on the parts of Behring and Roux which had finally led to the great triumph. The point made was that diptheria antitoxin was not a chance discovery but the result of patient and laborious laboratory work in which the fundamental biological principles had been applied. The suggestion presented was that what was needed to solve many of the other great problems in medicine were men and resources which could be devoted solely to the work of research." [Duffus and Holt 1940:138]

After this initial conversation, Rockefeller, Jr. held several more informal interviews with Holt. These conversations culminated in a dinner at Holt's house in March, 1901 at which Dr. Christian A. Herter was also present. Herter was a wealthy physician who was interested in research and had set up a laboratory in his own house to do his work. Herter was also a family friend being the neighbor of Rockefeller, Sr. at his summer home on Mount Desert Island. According to one account of the meeting, the two men were told of the investigations being made by Murphy into medical schools in the United States and foreign research institutes. Rockefeller, Jr. asked: "Suppose my father were to give $20,000 a year for ten years. What would you do with it to promote medical research?" (Nevins 1940:472). This triggered a detailed discussion that ended with Rockefeller, Jr. asking the men to name other physicians who might be interested in directing such an enterprise. The first name mentioned by both men was William H. Welch, who had been their professor while they were students at Bellevue Medical College before Welch went to Johns Hopkins. They also named Herman Biggs, Director of the New York City Department of Health; Theobald Smith of Harvard, and T. Mitchell Prudden of Bellevue (Fosdick 1956:113). Holt recalled that Rockefeller said: "We don't know these other gentlemen, but we do know you, and you can serve as a medium of connection between our family and the medical men you have suggested as advisors" (Corner 1965:32). On March 15, 1901 Herter wrote to Welch to tell him of the events that had transpired at the dinner meeting. He asked Welch to serve on the advisory board, adding: "Mr. Rockefeller has expressed a strong wish that you serve on the Advisory Board and would be much gratified if you could see your way clear to acting as its Chairman. ... While Mr. Rockefeller's interest in the establishment of a research laboratory is primarily humanitarian rather than scientific, I am confident that he would never allow his desire for practical results to hamper the laboratory in its direct or indirect efforts to obtain such results." [Flexner and Flexner 1966: 273]

In this same letter, Herter mentioned that the institute, as conceived at that point in time, was to be extremely modest, having to prove itself before it would receive a large endowment. He also named several other prominent researchers who could possibly serve on the advisory board. Welch agreed to serve on the Board but begged off being made Chairman as he was pressed for time. He also wrote to Rockefeller, Jr. expressing his willingness to "cooperate in every way in my power."

The Association of American Physicians (AAP) was an off-shoot of the American Medical Association (AMA) composed of elite scientific physicians who wanted meetings to deal with research reports rather than internal AMA politics. All of the people who had been considering a research institute were present at the annual meeting of the AAP held at the Arlington Hotel in Washington, D.C. in early May, 1901. During this meeting, the ideas and plans were discussed by the physicians and the meetings ended with Welch being asked to write to Theobald Smith of Harvard asking him to take on the Chairmanship. The letter, dated May 5, 1901 read in part: "The proposition now made by Mr. Rockefeller is to give twenty thousand dollars annually for at least 10 years, and place in the hands of the committee the arrangements for its expenditure" (Flexner and Flexner 1941: 274). This had been formally notified in a letter from Rockefeller, Sr. to Holt on April 29, 1901. Although Welch himself favored the affiliation with a university he noted:

"It seems that Mr. Rockefeller is more favorable to the proposition of making use of the new laboratory ... [of] the New York City Board of Health ... with the understanding that we shall be entirely independent. . . . I do not think that it is worthwhile to discuss any other place for the laboratory except in New York, and indeed that is probably the most suitable location."

Two things occurred that changed the picture presented above. Rockefeller, Jr. felt very strongly about having Welch as the Chairman of the institute, although they had not as yet met, and it was decided to delay the establishment of a laboratory and to give out grants to existing researchers. This being the case, Smith was dropped from consideration as Director and Welch consented to become the Director of the Institute. The initial board of the Institute was then composed of Welch as President; Prudden as Vice-President; Holt as Secretary; Herter as Treasurer, Herman Biggs, Theobald Smith, and Simon Flexner.

The first meeting of the new Institute was held on May 25, 1901 during which a discussion was held regarding the disbursement of the first year's funds. Although they had $20,000 to distribute, they could only find $13,200 worth of promising research in 1901 and $14,450 in 1902 in grants ranging from $300 to $1,200 (Flexner and Flexner 1966: 274–76).

On June 4, 1901 the Institute was formally incorporated as the Rockefeller Institute for Medical Research. The popular and medical press reaction was wholly favorable.

Major New York papers of the day, the *Times*, *Tribune*, and the *Evening Post* all printed full accounts of the Institute in their June 2, 1901 editions with editorials. Corner believed that Prudden had informed the editorial boards of the papers regarding the intentions of the Institute (Corner 1965: 44). The *Evening Post* editorialized:

"The American medical profession have been criticized for lack of original work. The new institute will provide for the release from cares of men of trained scientific intelligence, who will be enabled to devote themselves to the solution of definite problems." [Corner 1965: 38]

The *Times* wrote:

"The new institution is to be wisely and conservatively managed. It begins its operations without flourish of trumpets and in an unpretentious way. It spends its funds in directions that seem to offer the best prospects of immediate results. Nobody can promise sensational discoveries of momentous value at any particular time. The directors of the Rockefeller Foundation [sic] may hope for them, but they intend now to attack certain definite problems pressing for solution, and to let fame come to their new establishment when it has won it. They may at some future time see their work grow to be a great landmark in medical science, like that of the Pasteur Institute in Paris. But they are scientific men working in the scientific spirit and that spirit is not concerned with impressing the multitude." [Corner 1965: 38]

The medical journals also treated the new institute as a welcome development:

"The most important medical news of the month is perhaps the foundation of the Rockefeller Institute for Medical Research ..." [*Maryland Medical Journal*, June, 1901: 324]

"The generosity of Mr. John D. Rockefeller has established an institute to be known as the Rockefeller Institute for Medical Research. ... The potential value of an institution of this kind, and under such auspices, to medical science and to the interests of humanity can hardly be over-estimated." [*New York Medical Journal*, June 15, 1901: 1047]

"That he [John D. Rockefeller, Sr.] has seen fit to set aside a considerable sum of money for the advancement of medical science in this country will be hailed with universal approbation. We hope that his example may not long remain isolated, but that other wealthy men with liberal tendencies may find medicine and medical institutions, hitherto somewhat neglected, worthy objects for their generosity ... it is certainly encouraging and stimulating to learn that Mr. Rockefeller has become a patron of scientific medicine." [*Journal of the American Medical Association*, June 8, 1901: 1630].

"Such an institution as the one proposed has long been a necessity in this country. ... The example set by Mr. Rockefeller will be followed, doubtless, by rich men in other American cities, and a new era, it is hoped, will dawn for medical research on this side of the Atlantic." [*Medical Record*, June 8, 1901: 907]

In addition to the commentary in its journal, the AMA passed the following resolution at its annual meeting in St Paul, Minnesota (June 4-7, 1901):

> "Whereas Mr. John D. Rockefeller of New York, appreciating the great importance and humanitarian utility of pure scientific medical research, has recently donated the sum of $200,000 for the promotion of original investigation and has placed the control of the sum in the hands of a committee composed of representative medical scientists under the able chairmanship of Professor William H. Welch of Baltimore. Be it resolved that the medical profession represented by this American Medical Association desires to express profound appreciation of this generous gift. The gratifying fact that the importance and need of research and medicine are so clearly realized by the gentlemen. Also its wise selection of the committee having charge of the same. Be it further resolved that the secretary of the AMA be instructed to transmit a copy of these resolutions to Mr. Rockefeller." [Rockefeller Family Archives, Educational Interests]

The medical journals seemed far more interested in the potential of the Rockefeller largesse to open the door for other philanthropists looking for new vehicles for their giving. This potential was quickly realized. By December, 1901 the McCormick family of Chicago (and International Harvester), who were related to the Rockefeller family through marriage, were inquiring of the Rockefellers as to how they operated the Rockefeller Institute. On December 18, 1901 Harold McCormick wrote to his brother-in-law, Rockefeller, Jr. and asked:

> "It occurs to us that as the work which we are interested in seems to be on so nearly parallel lines with that which you have undertaken that we might be able to profit to the advantage of our institution by the experience which you have had in this connection. This information will presumably be in the direction of control or the degree of control which you hold over the future policies of the Institution, your relation to the Institution through its charter and to the board of directors." [Rockefeller Family Archives, Educational Interests]

On December 20, 1901 Harold McCormick replied to Rockefeller, Jr.:

> "I want to thank you for your supplementary telegram in answer to my question about your having control over the board of directors of

the medical institute. You covered the situation entirely by using the words 'technically the donor has no control over the board.' This is what we were after and it will assist us materially in reaching our conclusions..." [Rockefeller Family Archives, Educational Interests]

The result of these conversations was the creation of the John Rockefeller McCormick Institute for the Study of Infectious Diseases in Chicago in 1902 (Hirsch 1966: 84). It should be recalled that the McCormick family pediatrician was L. Emmett Holt and it is to be assumed that he gave the McCormicks the same speech he had given to Rockefeller, Jr. on the train ride from Cleveland. The institute was named for a young McCormick who died of an infectious disease in 1901 (Corner 1965).

Despite the public and professional tribute to the creation of the Rockefeller Institute, few people were happy with its operation. Gates thought it to be a waste of his idea; Rockefeller, Jr. thought it too conservative; and the Board of Directors who had opted for the grant award approach soon realized the error of their ways. A massive document was prepared entitled "Important Recommendations of the Directors of the Rockefeller Institute for the years 1901–1902". This work contained a review of the year's work and a proposal for expansion:

"Out of between 50 and 60 applications for aid in the prosecution of special researches, 23 were selected as of highest promise. These researches were such as could not be undertaken at all or would be greatly hampered without assistance. The directors have secured counsel in these selections from the heads of departments and others in the universities of Harvard, Yale, Johns Hopkins, Pennsylvania, Columbia, New York, Chicago, Wesleyan, Michigan, McGill, California and Western Reserve, and in many of these institutions work has been prosecuted. ... The directors however are united in the conviction that the highest aims of the institute cannot be secured in this way alone. Useful as such individual studies are and important as it is to enlist aid and to maintain the interest of research workers in established institutions of learning, it is not possible to secure the unity of aim and the coordination and mutual stimulus and support which are essential to the highest achievements in research. These are to be secured, we believe, only by the centralization of certain lines that leads to the work of the institute under a competent head or series of heads of departments in a fixed place with good equipment and a permanent endowment. The importance of unity of aim and coordination of work in research is obvious and the attempts which the institution might, we think, wisely make to discover the cause of such scourges as smallpox, measles, hydrophobia, and others of this group of diseases which are as yet wholly unknown. In these attempts it will be necessary to bring to bear on a single aim the resources of various phases of research, chemical, bacteriological, morphological and the prospects of success will be much greater if these related lines of study can go hand in hand. The largest measure of suffering and misery and the most serious mortality are gathered about the diseases of the lungs. These diseases, we believe, could be in large measure prevented if more accurate knowledge of their modes of acquirement were available and could be widely diffused among all classes of the community. Here also comprehensive researches along many lines can alone promise the best results ..." [Flexner and Flexner 1966: 281–82]

The argument continued for cancer and then the directors presented their recommendations calling for a well-equipped, well-endowed institute in New York, with an attached hospital. The institute would be organized departmentally, with heads of departments and assistants and research fellows and a large staff of technicians, janitors, maids, etc. As a starting point, the work of the institute should at first crystallize around the infectious diseases. The recommendations, it can be seen, do not vary very greatly from the original suggestions sent to Seth Low by Welch and Prudden in 1900. What is interesting is the way in which Rockefeller, Jr. got his father to approve the recommendations. He sent the recommendations to his mother and said:

"I am sending you herewith a copy of the report and recommendations of the Directors of the Rockefeller Institute, upon which report their decision as to the wisdom of building a laboratory in New York and effecting a permanent organization here was based. This report is the result of the united efforts of the various members of the board and of their earnest and most careful thought and study. It covers this situation so admirably that I feel sure you will enjoy reading it, and I am sending it to you hoping that you will sometime find father willing to let you read it aloud to him. There is no hurry about it or no real need of his reading it at all, except that I feel it would put him in closer touch with the work and give him a better idea of the careful way in which the men in charge are proceeding, also of the possibilities which the work has." [Fosdick 1956:113-14]

This is, in fact, not an isolated instance of this type of behavior on Rockefeller, Jr.'s part. He saw himself as the go-between between Gates and his father; Gates was the thinker and Rockefeller, Jr.'s job was to sell his father the ideas so he would financially back them. Rockefeller, Jr. did not himself control large sums of money until after his father died in the late 1930s.

In the midst of all this, Starr Murphy was continuing his research on medical schools and medical research institutes in the United States and Europe. In 1900, Harvard Medical School had found itself a new location and was seeking large amounts of money to endow a new medical school and several buildings. J.P. Morgan gave $1,185,000 to the cause (Harrington 1905:1389).

Since at that time it was still the majority opinion of people involved in the proposed institute (except Gates) that the institute should be affiliated with a university, Columbia and Harvard had been extensively researched by Murphy and at one time, it seems that the institute came very close to being affiliated with Harvard. In September, 1901 Harvard applied to Rockefeller, Sr. to become the home of the Rockefeller Institute. Murphy was sent up to explore the situation. On September 13, 1901 he wrote to Rockefeller, Jr.:

> "I went to Boston Monday afternoon and returned Wednesday night. The proposed enlargement of the medical school includes a considerable provision of medical research and in reaching a conclusion with regard to their request, it is well to consider the relation to the work of your own institute. I am not informed as to the later developments in connection with the latter institute. I would be obliged if you could refer me to the man who would know the most about it." [Rockefeller Family Archives, Educational Interests]

Rockefeller, Jr. put Murphy in touch with Welch, and when Murphy submitted his report on Harvard he included a section called "What would be the relations between the work of the Harvard Medical School as enlarged by the proposed plan and the Rockefeller Institute for Medical Research?"

"I had an interesting talk with Dr. Welch on this subject. He feels that the work at Harvard would not in any way interfere with the work of the Institute for Medical Research, but on the contrary would supplement and fit into it. He said that he did not consider that Harvard was proposing to give too much attention to research for a medical school, for the reason that men of reputation as investigators were an inspiration to students. He considered that high-grade schools of this character were necessary to furnish the men who are to do work in the Institute, and that the Institute should not be hampered with general teaching. He also expressed the opinion that considering the future development the proposed buildings would not be too large.

"My own feeling with regard to it is that the Institute will eventually form the crown of medical research in this country. A great deal of research is being done in the hospitals, but this is necessarily limited in its character by the purpose for which hospitals are created. ... The medical schools extend the scope of their research work considerably beyond that of the hospitals. ... And finally, above them all should come the work of your Institute for Medical Research which would take up the problems where the medical schools leave them, and treat them in their broadest aspects, and thus the hospitals and the medicals schools so far as they carry on research work, will lead it to and be feeders for the Institute, which will be the crown of the whole system." [Harrington 1905:1190–195]

Based on this report, Rockefeller, Sr. gave $1 million to Harvard in 1902.

On March 15, 1902 Nicholas Murray Butler wrote to Rockefeller, Jr., informing him that Columbia was looking for $3 million for its medical school. Rockefeller, Jr. responded on March 19, 1902 by saying:

"While my father might be willing after investigation, to join with others, he himself making a modest gift to the medical department of the university, I feel confident that in any event he will not feel inclined to contribute so large as you have suggested. Since you have requested, I will ask Mr. Starr J. Murphy, 115 Broadway, who represents us in educational matters, to make a study of the College of Physicians and Surgeons at his convenience after which I will bring the matter to my father's attention. That there may be no misunderstanding, allow me to emphasize that the making of this investigation does not in any way commit my father to a favorable consideration of your request. It is simply the means which we currently employ to get data on which he can base his judgments." [Rockefeller Family Archives, Friends and Associates]

He later wrote back to Butler on May 5, 1903 informing him:

"You wrote me desiring to call my father's attention to the needs of the medical department of Columbia University, in the hope that he might be inclined to make a gift to that department. I beg to say that after carefully considering the situation my father is not prepared to favorably consider the request."

During 1902, after the recommendations of the directors of the Institute were circulated, the reorganization began to pick up speed. There were several external reasons for this. Andrew Carnegie had just given $10 million to found the Carnegie Institution of Washington. Since the Carnegie Institution's charter was very broad, the Rockefeller organization was afraid that it would take in medicine and medical research as well, thus stealing the Rockefeller's thunder. To be sure, the two philanthropists were in competition with one another, or perhaps more accurately, their staffs felt they were in competition. The extent of the threat that the Carnegie Institution posed was so great that Rockefeller, Jr. talked to Carnegie and asked him to stay away from medical research, which Carnegie agreed to do (Rockefeller Institute Archives, May 14, 1902). There were also other rich entrepreneurs interested in getting into medical research. Plans were under way for the creation of the Phipps Institute for the Study of Tuberculosis in Philadelphia, and the McCormicks were starting to put together the McCormick Institute. Thus, for there to be any real publicity value in the Institute, Rockefeller had to really move on with the project. On June 13, 1902 Rockefeller, Jr. told his father that there was a need for $5 million in capital funds, but an immediate need for a million. Rockefeller, Sr. replied:

"As you so earnestly recommend, you may pledge one million dollars to be distributed throughout the next ten years. If if were left as you suggest, to be drawn at the option of the board, they might take a large portion in the early part of the ten years. We cannot say anything about five millions now." [Corner 1965: 52]

With the money firmly assured, the Board had now to find a fulltime Director. All the present members of the Board were young, mostly in their thirties and forties. All, with the exception of Smith, had had some amount of study or training in Germany. All were bacteriologists and used bacteriologic methodology and concepts in their work, different as that may have been. Welch's first choice for the job was Theobald Smith, who had recently accepted a position at Harvard (Flexner and Flexner 1941: 280). Smith declined the job and Welch's next choice was his former student, then Professor of pathology at the University of Pennsylvania, Simon Flexner. Flexner, under much pressure from Welch, eventually agreed to take the job, and went off to Europe to study how the Institutes there were set up and to acquire a library for the Rockefeller Institute. Flexner's salary at the Institute was to be $10,000 per year, his formal employment to begin on July 1, 1903 (Flexner and Flexner 1966: 281–83). With the directorship settled, there remained only the issue of affiliation to be reconciled. Although an affiliation with a university had been indicated as the likely outcome since the beginning, it was clear that the Rockefeller people had second thoughts about it. Gates was clearly against it, seeing the problems that emerged when a university bureaucracy was involved, rather than having direct control over the Institute. In addition, to affiliate the Institute with a university with an allopathic medical school would again, as in Chicago, bring objections from Rockefeller, Sr. It was therefore decided to keep the Institute independent and to buy land in New York City. The land was purchased in 1903 and in 1903–04 the plans for the Institute were drawn up. The Rockefeller Institute laboratories were officially dedicated in 1906.

In the Rockefeller Institute, the ideas and germinal discussions that had started out with the Rush–Chicago merger attempts began to take root. There was still wide disagreement on what scientific medical research should study and how and who should perform it, but the start was made with a research institute free from the constraints of university bureaucracy.

6
Gates and Medicine

In his autobiography, Gates made it clear that while the inspiration for the Rockefeller Institute was his, the way the Institute started off was not. He described the first few years of the Institute in the following scathing paragraph in his autobiography:

"Being preoccupied with other things, I introduced to Mr. Rockefeller [Jr.] a legal friend of mine, Mr. Starr J. Murphy, of Montclair, as qualified, though personally unacquainted with medicine, to make extensive inquiries of medical men in New York, Baltimore, Philadelphia and Boston respecting the feasibility of the proposed institute. The conclusions of the medical men were disappointing. Instead of the institute I advocated, they suggested that Mr. Rockefeller give a small sum, I think it was Twenty Thousand Dollars per year for ten years to selected individual laboratory workers in various parts of the country. The plan proved utterly futile. It was not until after several years of the complete failure of their system of scattered subventions that the medical gentlemen ventured timidly to organize an institute of research and give it a local habitation and a name ..." [Gates 1977:183]

The early development of the Rockefeller Institute was clearly different from the direction Gates had envisioned and did not reflect his perception of the potential of scientific medicine. The following analysis is based upon and distilled from the corpus of Gates's writing between the period under discussion and Gates's autobiography in 1928.

Gates and Medicine

By the late 1890s, Gates was much more a capitalist than a minister. He was on the Board of Directors or the President of several corporations including the Western Maryland Railroad, Colorado Fuel and Iron, Davis Coke and Coal Co., American Ship Building Corp., and American Linseed Oil Co. In addition, Gates was putting together the Mesabi iron ore range complex in Minnesota for the Rockefeller organization (Nevins 1953: 197–215). Gates considered himself to be a capitalist and certainly had a capitalist perspective on events. According to his autobiography, he had been making $2,500 a year as Secretary of the American Baptist Education Society. His salary was raised to $4,000 when he joined Rockefeller in 1891. By 1902, he was making $30,000 yearly (at age forty-one), had saved $60,000, and had over $500,000 invested in stocks and bonds (Gates 1977:145–46). In some ways, though, Gates was very different from the capitalists of his period. Because of the way he became a capitalist, that is through joining Rockefeller's organization rather than the long arduous process of capital accumulation or through inheritance, his views on society were clearly different. He was, what is called today, a corporate liberal, a capitalist who tried to ameliorate class struggle by sacrificing accumulation to increase stability (Weinstein 1968). This can be clearly seen from an undated and unpublished memorandum Gates wrote entitled "Capital and Labor":

> "The real fight is this: Shall labor have more and capital have less? Let us remember that is an absolute see-saw. The plank between them is stiff. If labor goes up, capital comes down; if capital goes up, labor comes down. There are no two ways about it. It is impossible, utterly impossible, unthinkable, unimaginable, that labor as a whole can have increases of wages except capital as a whole shall have a decrease of interest and rent. ... I am inclined to think that the thing that labor asks, namely, a large share at the expense of capital is, on the whole, for the public good, and that capital had better be content with one percent, two percent or three percent and give the balance to labor; that the world will be happier and wiser, a better and more comfortable place for us all to live in, and human suffering reduced, if that can be brought about." [Gates Papers, Rockefeller Foundation Archives]

What is especially significant about the above comments is not just the identification of capital and labor as eternal enemies, a perspective which Gates probably picked up in his studies of political economy in college, but the solution which Gates proposes for the problem. Rockefeller, Sr. did not share that perspective, nor did most of the other people with whom Gates associated at the Rockefeller philanthropies. Nevertheless this provides an insight into the inner Gates who was reflective about the problems around him even if he didn't act on those reflections.

At the time that Gates was reading Osler's *Principles and Practice of Medicine*, the social stability of the United States was tenuous. Despite the defeat of William Jennings Bryan the candidate of Populism in the Presidential election of 1896, rural agrarian disaffection and urban immigrant problems combined with a rapidly growing labor movement in the United States led many to search for a peaceful alternative; a way of restoring or creating a national harmony and unity that would not, at the same time, disrupt the dominant mode of social relations. In reading a long and fairly dense medical textbook, Gates saw that alternative as scientific medicine. Gates saw in medicine not just a means of improving health but a means of ameliorating class struggle.

Gates was able to read much into scientific medicine because his definition of disease was extremely wide, far wider than that of the scientists who were studying medicine. On several occassions, Gates outlined his own definition of disease which encompassed a broad range of social and political issues. He stated:

> "Disease is the supreme ill of human life and it is the main source of almost all other human ills, poverty, crime, ignorance, vice, inefficiency, hereditary taint, and many other evils." [Gates 1923:16–17]

and:

> "... disease is a prolific root of every conceivable ill, physical, economic, mental, moral, social. Disease, the physical pain and anguish it produces in the sick, the agony of heart in parents, children, friends, the fear of it, and the dread of it—disease with its attendant evils is undoubtedly the main single source of human misery. And the great mass of the charities of the world concern themselves directly or indirectly with relieving or mitigating such evils and miseries of

society as are due mainly to disease." [Gates 1977:186]
and:

> "Another of our habitual themes [talked about in the Gates household] is that the evils of society are not fundamentally economic but are physical and moral. They are to be cured by improvement in the public health and in the public morals and not fundamentally by economic readjustments which at best will be secondary and remote in their effect on the world's progress." [Gates to C.W. Eliot, November 1, 1910, Gates Papers, Rockefeller Foundation Archives]

The viewpoint expressed by Gates in these quotes reflects an ideology which holds that while problems seen as social require a political solution, problems seen as scientific need only a technical solution. People were not unhealthy because of the system of production under which they labored and the relations of production engendered by that system, rather they were sick because of germs, which could be identified and eliminated. According to Gates, it was not industrial capitalism, the trusts, or rapacious greed that were problems as the socialists and other dissidents in society maintained; it was in fact capitalism that would find a cure for all disease and lead to a happier and healthier society.

Gates's understanding of disease and disease etiology was based on a simplistic understanding of the germ theory of disease. Gates was, however, by no means alone in this understanding.

A brief digression on the germ theory of disease

It is necessary to digress briefly to discuss the development of the germ theory of disease.

Prior to the mid-nineteenth century, theories of disease origin varied between disease as direct punishment from God for improper behavior to disease as a result of filth or unclean living. While theories of disease as caused and spread by biological agents dated as far back as the sixteenth century, the inability to see bacteria and the lack of a methodology to prove causation gave these theories little credence.

In mid-nineteenth-century Europe, two major theories of

A System of Scientific Medicine

disease origin were in open competition. Contagionism held that disease was spread by commerce and population movements while Anti-contagionism postulated that disease was not contagious but sprang from miasmas, clouds of decaying matter activated by certain meteorological conditions. It is noteworthy that these theories were debated politically and ideologically as well as scientifically. Ackerknecht (1948: 567) noted:

> "Contagionism was not a mere theoretical or even medical problem. Contagionism had found its material expression in the quarantines and their bureaucracy, and the whole discussion was thus never a discussion on contagion alone, but always on contagion and quarantines. Quarantines meant, to the rapidly growing class of merchants and industrialists, a source of losses, a limitation to expansion, a weapon of bureaucratic control that it was no longer willing to tolerate, and this class was quite naturally with its press and its deputies, its material, moral and political resources behind those who showed that the scientific foundations of quarantine were naught, and who anyhow were usually sons of this class. Contagionism would, through its associations with the old bureaucratic powers, be suspect to all liberals, trying to reduce state interference to a minimum. Anticontagionists were thus not simply scientists, they were reformers, fighting for the freedom of the individual and commerce against the shackles of despotism and reaction."

The anti-contagionist theory was particularly amenable to expansion. It was not a difficult transition from believing that disease was caused by deleterious natural conditions to believing that there was a social component to those conditions as well. The sanitary movement with its focus on clean water supplies and filtered sewerage systems were products of anti-contagionist theory. There were also radical anti-contagionists who founded the movement known as Social Medicine which looked at disease as primarily stemming from social exploitation and uneven living conditions. Rudolf Virchow, the leader of this movement, saw the role of the physician as the defender of the poor and saw the elimination of disease in social revolution. To this end he took up arms in the rebel barricades in Berlin during the revolution of 1848.

With the defeat of the revolutions in mid-nineteenth-century

Europe, the Social Medicine movement floundered. Its leaders were harassed and denied promising jobs and academic appointments. Medical research became outwardly less politicized as it was carried out primarily in the laboratory rather than in the streets.

In the 1870s and 1880s new developments in technology such as the oil immersion lens and staining reagents allowed for the visualization of bacteria under the microscope. From these developments flowed a germ theory of disease with a corollary theory of the specific etiology of disease. In essence, germ theory maintained that every disease was caused by a specific agent, a different bacterium. It implied that: 1) there were specific diseases that were caused by specific bacteria; 2) each bacterium could cause one and only one specific disease; 3) the actual cause of each disease was this specific microscopic biological agent; 4) a cure within the realm of biology existed—a predator, so to speak, that could destroy the infecting agent. Most simply stated, germ theory could be expressed as one germ = one disease = one cure (Berliner and Salmon 1978).

While germ theory was a major progressive step in the development of medicine, scientists of the time exaggerated the importance of specific etiology and neglected all that had been previously learned about the non-bacterial (e.g. social, environmental) factors in disease causation and spread. Rather than making the reasonable assumption that while bacteria were the prime causative agents of disease, their pathogenic effects were mediated socially and environmentally, physicians totally dismissed the non-biological factors. The conventional understanding of germ theory, as opposed to the scientific understanding, was similarly mechanical and reductionist as it was articulated toward the end of the nineteenth century.

Many explanations are possible for why the germ theory was understood in this way including: 1) over-enthusiasm on the part of bacteriologists, overwhelmed by the rapid accumulation of new knowledge; 2) political repression of alternative approaches; 3) simple ignorance of a dynamic process. Regardless of why this particular understanding emerged, the popular conception of germ theory was extremely conservative.

A System of Scientific Medicine

While earlier eras looked to individual moral failure for the cause of disease, the sanitary era looked to the external environment; Social Medicine looked to the class structure of society, and germ theory placed the responsibility for disease on an invisible and amoral microbe. When disease was thought to be caused by moral turpitude, the cure was in prayer and behavior reform; when it was thought to stem from pollution of the external environment, the cure lay in massive expenditures for clean water and sanitation systems; when it was caused by an oppressive social structure, the cure was in revolution and the overthrow of the existing social order. Germ theory, however, found its cure in research. Research did not require individual reform, massive investment, or social reorder.

The germ theory, as it developed, became consistent with and defensive of the social and political status quo. Germ theory was not the conscious creation of capitalists acting in their own self-interest—far from it. It did however fit well into the belief systems and institutions of capitalism. The mechanical and reductionist understanding of disease causation fostered by germ theory lent itself well to the industrial mentality of the time which lent further credibility to the theory in the eyes of philanthropically inclined entrepreneurs. Gates, for example, could describe the operation of the body to Rockefeller in the following way:

"It is interesting to note the striking comparisons between the human body and the safety and hygienic appliances of a great city. Just as in the streets of a great city we have 'white angels' posted everywhere to gather up poisonous materials from the streets, so in the great streets and avenues of the body, namely the arteries and the blood vessels, there are brigades of corpuscles, white in color like the 'white angels', whose function it is to gather up into sacks, formed by their own bodies, and disinfect or eliminate all poisonous substances found in the blood. The body has a network of insulated nerves, like telephone wires, which transmit instantaneous alarms at every point of danger. The body is furnished with the most elaborate police system, with hundreds of police stations to which the criminal elements are carried by the police and jailed. I refer to the great number of sanitary glands, skillfully placed at points where vicious germs find entrance, especially about the mouth and throat. The

Gates and Medicine

body has a most complete and elaborate sewer system. There are wonderful laboratories placed at convenient points for a subtle brewing of skillful medicines. There is a vast system of dispensaries, suitably located, and there is a great Physician, whom I shall call Doctor Nature, who has an office in every human organism, without exception, and who knows more about the cause and treatment of disease than all the doctors in the world put together. The fact is that the human body is made up of an infinite number of microscopic cells. Each one of these cells is a small chemical laboratory, into which its own appropriate raw material is constantly being introduced, the processes of chemical separation and combination are constantly taking place automatically, and its own appropriate finished product being necessary for the life and health of the body. Not only is this so, but the great organs of the body like the liver, stomach, pancreas, kidneys, gall bladder are great local manufacturing centers, formed of groups of cells in infinite numbers, manufacturing the same sorts of products, just as industries of the same kind are often grouped in specific districts." [Gates 1911: 2 Rockefeller Foundation Archives]

When Gates read Osler's book that fateful summer he learned that:

"... besides the catching disease, there are 78 diseases of the digestive organs, 37 of the respiratory tract, 34 of the circulatory system, 15 of the blood stream, 27 of the kidneys, 106 of the nervous system. This list omits diseases of the eye, ear and skin. Nor does Osler enter the field of surgery.... When Osler's first edition appeared ... he was able to name a certain cure for only 5 diseases." [Gates 1923: 16–17]

he also learned that:

"Then there are numbers of diseases and illnesses, sometimes chronic and long continued, sometimes very short and amounting to nothing more than a temporary inconvenience, that are caused by germs multiplying in the digestive tract. They manifest themselves by headaches, by indigestion and by various derangements of the bowels and intestines. The study of these germs has been the special province of the present head of the Pasteur Institute. He has written several books upon the subject, two of which I have read. He shows that it is these poisonous germs in the intestinal tract that poison the blood and cause the hardening of the walls of the arteries which produces old age and all the symptoms of old age, and he believes that if we could clean out entirely the digestive tract from all germs, men would live ordinarily from twenty to forty years longer than they do; indeed, he fixes the normal limit of human life at one hundred and twenty years and believes that it is reduced to eighty mainly because of these poisonous germs." ['Notes on Homeopathy' 1, April, 1911, Letter to John D. Rockefeller, Sr., Rockefeller Foundation Archives]

Thus, when Gates read Osler's book, he saw a vast open field for philanthropy. All that was needed was money to support research which would uncover the causes (i.e. germs) of all the illnesses that harmed mankind. Since Gates believed that many of the more pressing problems of the day—ignorance, vice, poverty, crime, etc. were actually illnesses, their cure would lead to the strengthening of the social order. Gates thought that the source of societal problems was not the economic situation but physical ailments. His position was, as noted earlier, that these were "to be cured by improvements in the public health and public morals and not fundamentally by economic readjustments which at best will be secondary and remote in their effect on the world's progress."

In addition to the social reasons for pursuing such research, economic justification existed as well. Gates noted that "a recent report states that 20 per cent of the employees of all large establishments are always at home sick" (Gates 1923:16). Thus Gates's interest in medical research was drawn not strictly from his simplistic understanding of the germ theory but from a broader understanding of the economic and social implications of disease. Gates also saw health as a marker for the progress of civilization. "Health is fundamental to every other element in the social organism. Health is the accurate index of social progress; and disease is a fixed limitation to social progress" (Gates 1923:19). Medicine, as seen by Gates, would become a new religion:

"I am now talking about the religion, not of the past but of the future, and I tell you that as this medical research goes on you will find out and promulgate as an unforeseen by-product of your work new moral laws and new social laws, new definitions of what is right and wrong in our relationships with each other. You will educate the human conscience in new directions and new duties. You will make it sensitive to new distinctions. You will teach nobler conceptions of our social relations and of the God which is over us all. You may be doing work here [Rockefeller Institute] far more important than you dream for the ethics and the religion of the future. Theology is already being reconstructed in the light of science, in the light of what you and others are doing in research, and that reconstruction is one of the most important of the services which scientific research is performing for humanity." [Gates 1916: 6–7]

If Gates were simply an eccentric minister who came to these thoughts by reading a textbook of scientific medicine, he would have been quite an amazing individual. That he was in a position to implement the ideas that he developed has made him far more significant and powerful. Many people were looking for new ways to save capitalists' money, and improved health was an obvious approach since it had the potential to influence so many areas in the economy. But Gates was not a simple-minded economic determinist promoting scientific medicine because it might be a more effective or efficient medicine, he saw in medicine a new way to understand society that not only justified his activities, but gave the activities in which he engaged a moral imperative.

Gates's work for the Rockefeller organization around the time of the creation of the Rockefeller Institute consisted of building up the organizational structure of an industry through the vertical and/or horizontal expansion of Rockefeller holdings in the industry and making those industrial units more efficient to achieve a higher return on investment. Thus when Gates began to think about the future Rockefeller Institute, he imagined it to be a highly integrated research factory, with a detailed division of intellectual labor similar to the productive system of division of physical labor in an industrial factory. He pictured the Rockefeller Institute as an intellectual "trust" with a centralization of research in a single operating plant and a vertical integration of all the pieces of that research. Gates intended to set a productivity standard determined not by the rate of return on investment or the bottom line of a corporate financial report but by the number of bacteria isolated and the number of cures effected. Obviously with this vision of a major research factory, Gates could not be satisfied with the initial formulation of the Rockefeller Institute as merely a grant-making organization.

Two distinct factors seem to have been responsible for the original structure of the Rockefeller Institute. They were: 1) Rockefeller, Jr. had only recently joined Gates on the Committee on Benevolence and Gates must have felt obliged to let him make some of the decisions. At the same time, the younger Rockefeller was probably concerned that he not fumble his first major assignment in philanthropy and thus chose a more conservative path. 2) The physicians who were meeting to determine how the Rockefeller Institute would develop understood that the small amount of money (by Rockefeller philanthropic standards) was just the tip of the iceberg—that once started, Rockefeller, Sr. would continue to pour ever-increasing sums into a project —as long as it met satisfactory investment criteria and as long as it was producing what it was supposed to produce. Thus the physicians may also have been afraid to jump right into this risky venture of establishing one major institute and also saw virtue in the conservative path of awarding separate grants to individuals. Gates simply waited until everyone was dissatisfied with the Institute's initial direction to step in and impose his own structure. So after a false start as a grant-awarding agency, the Rockefeller Institute was established along the lines originally conceived by Gates.

In his autobiography, Paul De Kruif who worked at the Rockefeller Institute during the early 1910s, gave a lucid description of the Institute in those early heady days:

"What a temple of science the Rockefeller Institute was! It gleamed, materially, in comparison to the department of bacteriology in the old Medical Building at Ann Arbor [where De Kruif had trained under Frederick Novy], that grubby den of research reeked of guinea pigs, white rats and rabbits. At the Rockefeller you did not smell the animals. They were brought to you from a beautiful animal house in the bowels of the Institute by a servant, a diener. . . . Here at the Rockefeller all was different. Lab servants washed the glassware and cooked the culture medium and if you had a well enough trained technician, he could even do your experiments for you. . . . The

shrine of science, the Rockefeller was an education to me; ... I'd climb the front steps of the Institute. Inside the door, a bust faced me. Of Hippocrates? or Leeuwenhoek? or Pasteur? No indeed. As was meet and proper, here was a sculpture of John D. Rockefeller, Sr., the greatest of all searchers for God's gold. 'We're paying you well, we're giving you every advantage, now come through with a discovery', old John D. seemed to exhort me through his thin lips.
... For all its lavish facilities, its endless apparatus, its technical knowhow, the Rockefeller Institute in 1920, at the end of some twenty years of existence, seemed to have fallen somewhat short of its glorious promise. As a shrine of research, the institute had had a curious origin. It had not blossomed out of a great discovery like that of Pasteur and his living vaccines, or like that of Robert Koch and his invention of a solid culture medium that had enabled the isolation and trapping of most of the deadly anthrax and TB microbes. ... The Reverend Mr. Gates put a challenge to his advisors. What was it that medical science lacked? Not brains, not curiosity, not Pasteur's wild boldness. No, not these, it was money it lacked. Such at least was Mr. Gates' insight. Given enough of the yellow metal, the moolah, you could buy the bricks and mortar, the microscopes, yes even the men; you'd find plenty of men if you paid them decently. Then you could organize all the facilities for grand researchers to discover the cures of those deaths lamented in his textbook by Dr. Osler. It was a vision, it was a natural. ... Soon after the take-off there seemed to be a stunning success, a new serum, evolved by Dr. Flexner and his minion, Dr. Jobling, to cure epidemic cerebrospinal meningitis. This remedy was reported to lower its mortality by many percent—statistically significant. Without controls. You did not need them. This vindicated the Gatesean hypothesis, so it seemed. It hinted that the medical unknown was like a slot machine: feed it enough gold pieces and you're bound to hit the jackpot of a cure. The sad thing was that Drs. Flexner and Jobling had not so much initiated as repeated the discovery. Two German researchers, Drs. Jochmann and Kruse, had been ahead of them. Such was the beginning of the Rockefeller Institute for Medical Research in the first decade of the brilliant new twentieth century. But yet, and alas, as the years wore on the hoped for parade of cures did not come off. Could it be that the slot machine had turned out to be a one-armed bandit stealing God's gold from Mr. Rockefeller? It is true that the hospital of the Rockefeller Institute in the century's second decade did bring forth serums against Types I and II and later many other types of lobar

pneumonia, not downing their death rates sensationally, but for all that, seemingly statistically significant. But still in the opening years of the 1920s citizens went on dying like flies from the great majority of the maladies which, said Dr. Osler, lacked a curative medicine. To Dr. Flexner, to the Reverend Mr. Gates, to Professor Welch this must have seemed baffling. All the factors for success were there: the bricks, the glass, the hands, the well-trained heads, the master directorial mind. Yet the hoped for scientific offensive against multiple deaths can hardly be said to have achieved a breakthrough; on wide fronts it can indeed have been said to have fizzled out. [Though, curiously, the public did not think so. To the man on the street, and to many a humble physician the Institute was and still remains the temple of medical research.]"   [De Kruif 1962:13-22]

It should be noted that De Kruif was asked to leave the Institute when he published an anonymous article critical of medicine and doctors in a popular magazine of the time. However, De Kruif was correct in his analysis of the way that Gates conceived of the research act. Gates saw medical research as similar to industrial production. You had a set of inputs (raw materials or, in this case, scientists and laboratory equipment) that went through a process (in this case bacteriological research) and emerged with an output (bacterial identification or vaccine). Gates understood medicine only in these mechanistic terms as did most people in America and Europe at this time. It was not that Gates's perception of medicine was different from the mainstream of medical perception at this time, rather it was strictly in accord.

Besides serving as an advanced center for research on scientific medicine, the Rockefeller Institute also served as a public relations vehicle for Rockefeller, Sr. From Ida Tarbell's *History of the Standard Oil Company* (1904) which exposed the manner in which the Rockefeller fortune was accumulated, through the tainted money scandal in which a Congregationalist minister returned a gift made by Rockefeller because he felt the money was tainted by the blood that was shed for Rockefeller to obtain it, through the Landis Decision in which a Federal judge fined Standard Oil for illegal practices, through the dissolution of the Standard Oil Trust, through the Ludlow Massacre in which the families and children of striking workers in a Rockefeller-owned company were killed by state militia, the Rockefeller name was continually abused and scorned by the media that was not directly controlled by Rockefeller interests. One of the major functions of the Rockefeller philanthropic efforts was to reverse the public stereotype of Rockefeller. Thus the Rockefeller organization went out of its way to picture Rockefeller, Sr. as a kindly man trying to help humanity rather than as a man who allowed widows to starve in his quest for more money and as the man who killed workers to prevent them from unionizing. That this was an effective strategy can be seen from the fact that at the height of the furore over the Ludlow Massacre, New York newspapers seriously suggested that Rockefeller be given a Nobel Peace Prize for setting up the Rockefeller Institute. The actual situation being that when Alexis Carrell won the Nobel Prize for work that he did at the Rockefeller Institute, the Hearst Press said that "Rockefeller deserved half a dozen such awards". The *New York Evening Journal* had already commented editorially:

> "All that has been said of Rockefeller's actions accumulating may be true, and—what is more probable—nine-tenths of it may be false. But this surely is true. Rockefeller uses his money for all the people. He is doing as an individual what the nation as a whole has not the intelligence to do. He considers himself a responsible custodian of the millions that he had dipped up from the golden stream of opportunity. And humanity will be better off because of his work when he shall have been dead ten thousand years. His dollars fight disease, man's enemies, and ignorance, man's greatest enemy." [Nevins 1940: 632]

An example of the conscious attempt to gain publicity for the Institute and thus indirectly for Rockefeller can be seen in the following exchange between Gates and President Eliot of Harvard:

> "Along the same line I [Gates] am moved to ask you if you can be of any service in any way; in securing, or helping to secure, for Dr. Flexner the Nobel Prize on account of his work in Cerebro-Spinal Meningitis. I am presenting the matter also to Dr. Welch. Dr. Flexner says they seldom give this prize until after work has been demonstrated for a number of years and it is known that it will stand, but surely Dr. Flexner's work in Cerebro-Spinal Meningitis, now

known all over the world and tested practically in every country in the world in thousands of cases, justifies action—certainly it is the most remarkable discovery in recent times." [November 1, 1910, Rockefeller Foundation Archives]

Eliot replied: "I should be delighted to help secure for Dr. Flexner the Nobel Prize, on account of his work on Cerebro-Spinal Meningitis" (November 9, 1910, Rockefeller Foundation Archives). It should be noted that Eliot had lost a son to the disease before Flexner's discovery. Despite this lobbying on behalf of Simon Flexner, he did not receive the Nobel Prize. Moreover, as De Kruif noted in the passage from his autobiography cited above, Flexner's discovery was not new and had not yet been subjected to controlled trials to test its actual efficacy. In a later anecdote, De Kruif repeated his position on the necessity of controlled research design:

> "One of my colleagues at the Rockefeller Institute—Dr. Rufus Cole, a gentle man who had been kind to me—had published an essay proposing the thesis that medicine had now developed so far that it could be looked on as an independent science, on a par with physics and chemistry. What a mental gaffe! While disease must be studied in a modern hospital, at the same time nothing should be left undone to cure the patient, wrote the eminent author. What a howler, what hooey, what a contradiction in terms! To study a disease, to get to know it, shouldn't the student abstain from interfering with the cause of disease he was looking for? How otherwise do you establish your base line? What had Pasteur done in his immortal experiment with the fifty-two sheep at Pouilly le Fort? He'd vaccinated only half of them and left the other half as controls and had left everything undone to save them; and they had died—*les temoins*, controls, Pasteur had called them—sad witnesses to the power of the vaccine to save the others. That was science. And had my eminent author of the essay done likewise? He had not. He ordered his pneumonia serum given to all patients so that not a single one would die per adventure the experimental serum might save. But without the serum that single one might have lived anyway. Who knew?" [De Kruif 1962: 38]

The search for public approval for the Rockefeller family as the leaders in the establishment of systematic medical research was a natural concern of those people (including Gates) whose responsibility it was to present a positive image of the family to the public. The search for the Nobel Prize was just one effort to gain such publicity for the Rockefellers.

The real irony in all this was that Rockefeller, Sr., who was winning so much praise, had so little to do with the Rockefeller Institute. Not only did he not believe in scientific medicine but he refused to be treated by scientific physicians. He also refused to go near the Institute which bore his name. Nevins tells of an instance in which the younger Rockefeller tried to get his father to inspect the buildings of the Institute, which the elder Rockefeller steadfastly refused to do (Nevins 1940: 479).

7
The Reform of Medical Education

As noted earlier, one of the elements of Andrew Carnegie's "Gospel of Wealth" was that a major area of philanthropic concern should be health and medicine:

> "We have another most important department in which great sums can be worthily used—the founding or extension of hospitals, medical colleges, laboratories, and other institutions connected with the alleviation of human suffering, especially with the prevention rather than with the cure of human ills ..." [Carnegie 1962: 40]

To be sure, donations to the fields of health and medicine had always been a large part of philanthropy, especially the endowment of hospitals. It is interesting to note that neither Rockefeller, Sr. nor any of the Rockefeller philanthropies gave money to hospitals because they did not want to institutionalize or honor what they considered to be the weak points of society. Moreover, the Rockefellers felt strongly that there were certain obligations incumbent upon a community which philanthropy should not supplement, medical care of the sick being a case in point.

Little money, however, had gone to medical research. Carnegie had made only a few gifts to medicine, but those were quite significant. One of Carnegie's first endowments established the first laboratory for pathology in the United States in 1884. Dr. Frederick Dennis, a social acquaintance of Carnegie's, asked him to endow a laboratory in an attempt to influence William H. Welch, the country's leading pathologist, to stay in New York. Welch had been invited to take a position with the soon to open Johns Hopkins Medical School in Baltimore. Carnegie was persuaded to give $50,000 to the laboratory, situated near Bellevue Hospital, and it became known as the Carnegie Laboratory (Winslow 1929: 60--1). While unsuccessful in keeping Welch in New York, the laboratory received distinction by sending American physicians to the Pasteur Institute to study rabies and rabies vaccination and by sending American children who had rabies to Paris for Pasteur's treatment (Wall 1970: 832). By March of 1909, Carnegie had given a total of $176,000 to the laboratory and on the twenty-fifth anniversary of its opening, Carnegie said: "This institution is one of my first children. I have not seen as much of it as I should have liked to, but I assure you that today has brought back all my original store of love for it, and I shall never forget that it is in the honored list of universities of America" (Winslow 1929: 223, 229).

Carnegie gave $120,000 to Koch for his institute of medical research in Berlin and a grant to Madame Curie for work on radiography. He also gave money to universities in Scotland for medical research. Yet medicine was not a major recipient of Carnegie's benevolence. There is evidence that Rockefeller's aides talked with Carnegie's aides and won an agreement that Carnegie would keep away from significant donations to medical research, as the following letter from Emmett Holt to Mitchell Prudden on May 14, 1902 indicates. The two men, among the founders of the Rockefeller Institute, were discussing the progress of the Institute. "He [Rockefeller, Jr.] had already talked with Mr. Carnegie regarding the prospects and scope of the Carnegie Institute and had been told by him that the Carnegie Institute did not wish to enter the medical field at all. This, I think clears the ground for the development of our institute." In addition, when Carnegie was solicited by supplicants from hospitals and medical schools, he would tell them: "That is Mr. Rockefeller's specialty. Go see him" (Wall 1970: 832).

It was, however, the Carnegie Foundation which was the first philanthropic foundation to be interested in the reform of medical education.

With the opening of the Johns Hopkins University School of

A System of Scientific Medicine

Medicine in 1893, medicine began to move into its scientific era in the United States. At first the philanthropic foundations were not involved but when they moved in, the changes they effected were enormous. Early foundation involvement in medical education took the form of money for capital improvements or for specified research requiring an endowment. This would include Carnegie's above noted gift of the pathology laboratory to Bellevue; Rockefeller, Sr.'s gift of $1 million to Harvard in 1901 for new research buildings for the medical school and his gift of $500,000 to Johns Hopkins Hospital after the 1904 Baltimore fire.

A qualitatively new approach to medical education was taken by the foundations beginning with the request for aid from McGill Medical School in Montreal. William Osler, an alumnus of McGill and former professor there, wrote to Gates asking that Rockefeller take care of his old institution. The relationship between Gates and Osler, author of *The Principles and Practice of Medicine* has already been discussed. Osler said:

"You have of course noticed the hard whacks which my old alma mater McGill has had in these two big fires. No doubt Sir William MacDonald, who built the Engineering Department, will restore it, but I am afraid from what I hear that the Medical Faculty has been hit very hard by the loss of their fine buildings. Do you think it would be possible to interest Mr. Rockefeller to the extent of a couple of hundred thousand dollars? It would mean everything to them and would really encourage a group of men who have been doing splendid work for the community." [Cushing 1949: 774]

Gates responded within a few days by asking Osler to get the Dean of the medical school to prepare a statement indicating what McGill had done in the way of research and what the extent of the losses were. Osler replied:

"I have asked the Dean of the Faculty to prepare a statement of the research work which has been carried on lately at McGill in medicine. I think you will be surprised at its extent and variety. An endowment of $500,000 would enable them to further extend and carry on this work. To rebuild a thoroughly modern fireproof building will take all the moneys available and leave them hampered sadly for this advanced work, which they are really prepared to do, so far as the personnel of the faculty is concerned ..." [Cushing 1949:774]

On May 28, 1907 Gates wrote to Emmett Holt, Secretary of the Rockefeller Institute, asking:

> "The only question which interests us here is this: Is the Medical School at McGill University a center of investigation so highly adapted and so important as to justify Mr. Rockefeller or to justify the Rockefeller Institute, if it had funds available for the purpose, in placing several hundred thousand dollars at the disposal of McGill to be exclusively devoted to investigation? ... You would confer a great favor upon us if you and your co-laborers could answer this question." [Flexner and Flexner 1966:286]

Holt presented this letter to the Board of Scientific Directors of the Rockefeller Institute at their meeting on June 13, 1907. The record in the minutes reads: "The secretary read a letter from Fred. T. Gates asking on behalf of Mr. Rockefeller for advice regarding an appeal from McGill University for funds in aid of its medical school." A subcommittee of the Board of Scientific Directors was formed with William Welch, Simon Flexner and perhaps one other member, although Welch was given the responsibility for preparing the reply.

Welch took the opportunity to go well beyond the small issue of aiding McGill and decided to consider "a broad policy of advancing in the most effective manner possible the advancement of medical knowledge" since this was "the main purpose of the institute and the controlling purpose of the founder in its establishment." The Institute should "not be indifferent to the conditions of education in our better medical schools and should not rest upon the assumption that the educational side can be safely left to take care of itself." He noted that the Institute itself had been made possible by the advances in medical education which preceded it (i.e., Johns Hopkins) and would continue to be dependent upon medical education for future staff:

> "What character of medical school is it desirable to aid in the expectation of advancing medical knowledge? We believe that such aid should be granted only to certain medical schools which possess the following characteristics. The school should be upon a university basis, an integral part of an important university, completely con-

trolled by the trustees of the university, the teachers being supported by salaries paid by the universities and not by a division of the fees of students. The school must already be in possession of laboratories which have been productive in research. It must be clear that the heads of these laboratories and the teaching staff in general are selected primarily for their demonstrated capacity to advance and stimulate research and to train young men to become independent investigators. ... The school should furthermore have advanced requirements for the matriculation of students, either a college degree or collegiate training in sciences fundamental to medicine such as physics, chemistry and biology, being required for admission."

Welch listed only Harvard, Columbia, Johns Hopkins, Western Reserve, University of Chicago, and in part McGill as satisfying these requirements at that time (leaving out state university medical departments). Welch thought that the best way to further scientific research in such institutions was by furnishing:

"permanent gifts of money, under certain well-defined conditions, to be used for construction or equipment of laboratories or endowment of laboratories or of chairs connected with them or the provision of opportunities for hospital clinics associated with laboratories. ... In every instance very careful investigation would be required to ensure the proper bestowal of such gifts and their utilization with the ultimate aim of improving the conditions for the promotion of medical science. It is believed that occasional grants for specific purposes could not be made to serve the same useful purpose as permanent endowment for it is only upon the assurance for the future that the proper organization and work of laboratories can be securely effected."

Welch then went on to describe the advantages to humanity which such gifts would bring. Welch noted that the directors of the Rockefeller Institute would be willing to advise the Rockefeller office on the most useful way of disposing of the funds to advance medical science. They would, he promised, "endeavor to exercise the same care and thought which they have hitherto given to the interests of the Institute." He concluded by saying:

"It is desired by the Directors before expressing a definite opinion upon the application of the McGill Medical School to learn how far the general policy of granting aid to medical schools along the lines

Reform of Medical Education

suggested in this statement meets the approval of the founder of the Institute and his advisers." [Flexner and Flexner 1966: 286-88]

No aid, incidentally, was given to McGill at that time. Osler, writing to a former colleague said: "I hear from Welch privately that the Rockefeller will not do anything for McGill at present toward the buildings, but that after everything is settled they may be prepared to make some endowment for research" (Cushing 1949: 775).

Simon Flexner, from an insider's position, stated that Welch was trying to use this situation to get the Rockefeller organization to take up large-scale support of medical education (Flexner and Flexner 1966: 288). By the time the Rockefeller philanthropies were prepared to get into the field, many of the preconditions for aid to medical schools that were listed by Welch had largely been met through dynamics occurring in medical education due to other foundations and other factors. The most important of these was the Carnegie Foundation and its Bulletin Number 4 —the Flexner Report.

The Carnegie Foundation

The Carnegie Foundation for the Advancement of Teaching was founded in 1905 with an endowment of $10 million. It was the first large-scale multimillion-dollar foundation established by Andrew Carnegie. Its original purpose was to grant retirement pensions to professors at American colleges and universities. Savage described how, as a trustee of Cornell University, Carnegie learned about the low salaries and near poverty existence of most college professors and he created the Carnegie Foundation to address this problem (Savage 1953: 30). The Board of Trustees of the Foundation consisted almost entirely of the Presidents of the leading institutions of higher education in the United States. The President of the Foundation was Henry S. Pritchett, former President of MIT. While Carnegie envisioned the purpose of the foundation to be the granting of pensions, Pritchett and the other trustees saw the foundation as a vehicle for promoting educational change. They decided that their first act should be to define exactly what a college was so that only professors from institutions that fit their definition would be eligible for a Carnegie pension. At the time there were over 1,000 institutions in the United States that identified themselves as colleges or universities. The Board's definition of an eligible college was:

> "An institution to be ranked as a college must have at least six professors giving their entire time to college and university work, a course of four full years in the liberal arts and sciences, and should require for admission not less than the usual four years of academic or high school preparation or its equivalent." [Smith 1974:100]

The requirement for six professors was interpreted to mean six distinct departments of instruction. To measure preparation for college, the Foundation developed the "Carnegie Unit", a measure of the amount of secondary school education by subject matter (Smith 1974:100). Having guaranteed the academic qualifications of the professors and the students, the institutions themselves had to demonstrate an endowment of over $200,000 and they were not permitted any religious affiliation in their charters (Hollis 1939:136).

It is important to note that none of these criteria was particularly original. The Carnegie Foundation was the first institution to pull these separate criteria together and coerce institutions into abiding by them. The method of coercion was solely the ability not to grant retirement pensions to the professors of the institution, a power that was to prove extremely persuasive. During the first year of operation of the Foundation only 52 colleges (out of 1,000 possible institutions) qualified for the Carnegie pensions.

With the criteria for colleges determined and the system for granting retirement pensions established, the Carnegie Board next turned its sights to professional education.

The American Medical Association Committee on Medical Education

The American Medical Association (AMA) was an organization trying to come to terms with medical education in the United States. Representing the university medical school scientist faculty and the practitioner elite in American medicine, the AMA attempted to raise the standards of medical education to a level that justified and affirmed their own individual investments in professional education. The AMA formed a Committee on Medical Education in 1904, and this committee performed a survey of medical education in 1906. The survey evaluated each medical school in the United States on a set of ten criteria and also by the number of students from each school who passed state licensing board exams. The results of the survey were never made public.

This medical educational campaign of the AMA actually met with considerable success in that many of the medical schools were restructuring themselves to become more integral parts of universities and upgrading their standards for entrance. The schools also demanded more preparation on the part of the students and offered an education more in line with the new developments of scientific medicine than they had previously. The AMA kept up its pressure though and its success can be seen in the fact that the organization increased from 8,400 members in 1900 to 70,000 members in 1910 (Berliner 1975).

At the third annual conference of the Council on Medical Education of the AMA held on April 29, 1907, Chancellor Kirkland of Vanderbilt University presented a paper entitled "Conditions Controlling General and Medical Education in the South". The speech, as recorded in the Minutes of the Council, included the following passage:

> "Twenty years ago, Vanderbilt University adopted the policy of discarding preparatory work, of rejecting preparatory students and placing conditions for entrance that were practically identical with those maintained in the first class institutions of the East. We did that in 1887 and reduced our students with one blow ... by about one half. We have sacrificed something for our faith in educational work; and yet, gentlemen, perhaps no one fact can bring before you more forcibly the general condition of things in the southern states than this, that in this year, 1907, twenty years after we have made our fight and twenty years after we have established our standard the Carnegie foundation for the advancement of teaching issued a bulletin defining the preliminary educational requirements necessary

A System of Scientific Medicine

for a high grade college in fourteen units, and the Carnegie Foundation for the advancement of teaching has caused a shudder to run through all these institutions in the South by the publication of that report. ... If this council would inspect and tell the truth about all our institutions, point out their defects, point to their equipment and give the facts as regards them, and as regards their manner of teaching, the moral force that would be exerted by such inspection would be a tremendous power and would have an uplift that could not be calculated or realized. That, sir, would be more efficient in the long run than an attempt by too drastic legislation to secure results that might work disaster to the cause we all have so dearly at heart. [loud applause]" [Minutes of the AMA Council on Medical Education 1907]

There is no direct connection between this speech and the subsequent cooperation between the Carnegie Foundation and the AMA. It does, nevertheless, give an indication of the effect of the Carnegie Foundation educational work in the South and has served as a proximate reason for closer work between the organizations.

8
Abraham Flexner and the Flexner Report

Abraham Flexner was born in Louisville, Kentucky, in 1866, one of nine brothers and sisters. His father was engaged in a merchant business until it folded during the recession of 1873. Flexner's oldest brother, Jacob, established a pharmacy and used the profits from that business to send Abraham to college. Abraham attended the Johns Hopkins University in Baltimore, Maryland, an institution with which he was to have much contact over the rest of his life. Hopkins had been founded in 1876 by Johns Hopkins, a Baltimore railroad entrepreneur (the Baltimore and Ohio Railroad), who endowed it with a gift of $7 million—the largest gift at that time ever made to a university in the United States. The money was to endow a university, a medical school and a hospital. The first President of the University, Daniel Coit Gilman, who had been involved with the Sheffield Scientific School at Yale, was an educational innovator and was determined to establish a new and progressive center for graduate education in the United States. Needing an undergraduate component to enable the institution to remain solvent, Johns Hopkins began accepting undergraduates in 1876. Abraham Flexner enrolled in 1883, and was able to graduate in just two years. The educational innovations, the lack of bureaucratic formality and the direct contact with the faculty gave Flexner a lifelong appreciation of Johns Hopkins University.

Upon graduation, family finances dictated that Flexner return to Louisville. He obtained a position in the Louisville high school teaching Greek and quickly became a popular and respected teacher. His ability to make progress with formerly incorrigible students led to requests from the local gentry that he tutor their sons (and occasionally daughters) so they could pass college admission examinations. In 1890 Flexner began to devote all his time to this activity and he continued for fifteen years. Mr. Flexner's School, as it was known, achieved some renown, even winning praise from President Charles Eliot of Harvard who noted in a letter to Flexner that students from his school matriculated at Harvard at younger ages than did students from other prep schools (Flexner 1960).

Flexner used the income generated through his school to help sustain the family pharmacy and to help his siblings earn advanced degrees. Of particular note is the fact that Simon Flexner, Abraham's older brother, had attended a proprietary medical school in Louisville and was working in the drug store. He was encouraged by Abraham to attend the new medical school just opening at Johns Hopkins in order to learn more about microscopy, his pet interest. Simon Flexner went to Hopkins in 1895 and stayed for ten years as an assistant to William Welch and later went on to become the first Director of the Rockefeller Institute and other Rockefeller medical philanthropic ventures.

Flexner had long been a believer in coeducation and his first female student, Anne Crawford, went to Vassar College and later returned to Louisville and married Abraham, her former teacher. She began a career as a playwright, becoming successful enough to allow Abraham to give up the responsibilities of teaching.

In 1905, Flexner started a Master of Education program at Harvard University in Cambridge, Massachusetts. At Harvard most teaching was done by graduate assistants and the formal bureaucracy was quite rigid, just the opposite of Hopkins. Flexner disliked Harvard intensely and left after a year to pursue research on the German educational system. In 1906, Flexner left for Germany and stayed there for two years. At the end of his stay he wrote a monograph *The American College* (1908) which was a critique of American higher education particularly as practised at Harvard. The book received little critical or popular recogni-

Abraham Flexner and the Flexner Report

tion and Flexner returned to the United States in 1908 without any firm plans for his career.

Flexner and the Carnegie Foundation

When Flexner returned to New York he was seeking a job. As he noted in his autobiography, he needed the money. While he may have been attracted by the name of the Carnegie Foundation for the Advancement of Teaching, he would probably have known that the agency was solely involved in granting pensions to retired professors at that time. It seems probable that Henry Pritchett, the President of the Carnegie Foundation, had broached the idea of a study of medical education with Simon Flexner or William Welch at the Rockefeller Institute and Simon may have suggested that Abraham consider working at the Foundation. Flexner's autobiography describes the initial meeting which has become something of a folk legend in medical educational circles:

> "It had occured to me that I might find congenial occupation at the Carnegie Foundation, and I asked President Remsen [of Johns Hopkins], Mr Gilman's successor, for a card of introduction to Dr. Pritchett. When I presented this introduction Dr. Pritchett allowed me to read a speech which he had written for delivery at Brown University and in which he had taken much the same line that was advocated in my little book. When I next saw him he asked me whether I would like to make a study of medical schools. As our family resources had been depleted during the preceding three years, I was, I confess, prepared to do almost anything of a scholarly nature; but it occurred to me that Dr. Pritchett was confusing me with my Brother Simon at the Rockefeller Institute, and I called his attention to the fact that I was not a medical man and had never had my foot inside a medical school. He replied, 'That is precisely what I want. I think these professional schools should be studied not from the point of view of the practitioner but from the standpoint of the educator. I know your brother, so that I am not laboring under any confusion. This is a layman's job, not a job for a medical man.'" [Flexner 1960: 70–1]

In another version of this story, from Flexner's biography of Pritchett, Pritchett said the following:

"What I have in mind is not a medical study, but an educational one. Medical schools are schools and must be judged as such. For that, a very sketchy notion of the main functions of the various departments suffices. That you or any other intelligent layman can readily acquire. Such a study as I have in mind takes that for granted. Henceforth these institutions must be viewed from the standpoint of education. Are they so equipped and conducted as to be able to train students to be efficient physicians, surgeons, and so on?" [1943:109]

While the need for this study to be conducted by Flexner may have been clear to Pritchett, the Board of the Carnegie Foundation was not completely convinced. Pritchett fought a hard battle to get the Board to accept Flexner for this job. In part the problem was that many of the Board members did not think that the Foundation should be studying the professions, that its function was solely to grant pensions to retiring college professors. Many apparently also thought that should there be a study, either a physician or a better known layman should be in charge. Pritchett is reported to have told Flexner: "I had to say [to the Board] that I must be free to choose my own associates, for whose competency I assume full responsibility. Your salary will be small, smaller than I like—$3,000 a year; but when you travel you will be supported by the Foundation" (Flexner 1943:110).

Pritchett, in fact, may have regretted his choice of Flexner for soon after Flexner embarked on his study, Pritchett was forced to write letters to several people that revealed some concern:

"Dear Dr. Councilman [William T. Councilman, Professor of Pathology at Harvard] Before asking Mr. Abraham Flexner to begin work here in connection with the study of professional education, I consulted a number of persons concerning his ability and character. Since he has begun work, however, a number of criticisms have come to me about him, generally in the way of casting some doubt upon his judgement and indicating somewhat erratic tendencies. There appears also to have been something at Harvard which caused friction. I shall appreciate it if you will give me confidentially a statement with regard to these matters, which shall go no further than myself . . ." [Berliner 1977:603–09]

A variant of that letter went: "Within the past few days, however, a good many criticisms have come to me concerning him, somewhat to the effect that he is erratic and hard to get along with and somewhat uncertain in his judgement . . . " (Berliner 1977:603–09). The only response to these inquiries still extant in the Henry S. Pritchett papers in the Library of Congress is from Dr. Councilman, who responded:

> "I have not known Mr. A. Flexner well, but I have liked what I have seen of him. I should think he might be somewhat erratic and probably hasty in judgement, but a very able and valuable man for all that. I think it is more or less easy to explain why he should not be a persona grata to many of the men at Harvard just at present, for his book criticized many of the conditions at the college, and I have never found that men take very kindly to criticism especially when it comes from the outside. While he was at Cambridge he lived with a rather erratic family and he worked with Munsterberg. I have not heard of any friction having developed while he was at Cambridge. He did not know a great many people there, but I have heard him very well spoken of by Munsterberg and others." [Berliner 1977:603–09]

It should be noted that negative comments such as these followed Flexner throughout his public life as is evidenced by this segment of a letter from Charles Eliot to Rockefeller, Jr.:

> "You are doubtless aware that negotiation in matters which divide opinion strongly is not Mr. Flexner's forte. He is a first rate man for inquiry, study and the devising of experiments, but in controversial matters he arouses strong opposition, partly I think by his aspect of eagerness and partly by a certain satirical humor." [Berliner 1977:603–09]

It is necessary to digress from this discussion of the making of the Flexner Report to describe the role of the AMA and its Council on Medical Education.

Sometime during 1908, the Council on Medical Education of the AMA wrote to President Pritchett of the Carnegie Foundation telling him of the work they were doing with educational reform and inviting him to come and talk with them (Flexner 1943:108). Pritchett was interested in the reform of the professions and, according to Flexner, suggested he had wanted to start off with reform of the legal profession but had encountered resistance from the American Bar Association. Pritchett was thus quite amenable to the friendly overtures from the AMA. He had to convince his Board of Trustees and the founder, Andrew Carnegie, that this was a worthwhile task, as they thought it well beyond the scope and realm of the Foundation's responsibilities (Flexner 1943:109). Carnegie himself was to say that the professional studies, in fact all the bulletins that the foundation produced, were interesting but clearly secondary to the main goal of providing pensions to teachers. Pritchett having finally secured the permission of his Board next had to find someone to conduct a study of medical education in the United States. This brings us back to Abraham Flexner.

From the beginning, it was clear that the study was to be conducted jointly with the Council on Medical Education of the AMA. We do not know from any published documents when Flexner first started to work on his project. It was probably during the late summer or fall of 1908. Flexner noted that he began by conducting a thorough literature review, being particularly impressed with Billroth's *The Medical Sciences in the German Universities*. He also went to Chicago to meet with the Secretary of the AMA, Dr. George H. Simmons, and to read the previous reports prepared by the Council on Medical Education. At the conclusion of this phase of the project, Flexner went to Baltimore to meet with the faculty of the Johns Hopkins Medical School. He wrote:

> "How fortunate for me that I was a Hopkins graduate!—where I talked at length with Drs. Welch, Halstead, Mall, Abel and Howell, and with a few others who knew what a medical school ought to be, for they had created one. I had a tremendous advantage in the fact that I became thus intimately acquainted with a small but ideal medical school embodying in a novel way, adapted to American conditions, the best features of medical education in England, France, and Germany. Without this pattern in the back of my mind, I could have accomplished little." [Flexner 1960:74].

It should be remembered at this point that a few years earlier Welch had been thinking about improving the system of medical education in response to Gates's invitation to the Board of the Rockefeller Institute, following the fire at McGill University. From the staff and directors of the Rockefeller Institute to whom Flexner had ease of access through his brother Simon and the Hopkins faculty, Abraham Flexner had a clear notion of how laboratory scientists felt medical education should be obtained.

The records of the Council on Medical Education document that the first meeting where the study of medical education was discussed occurred in New York on Monday, December 28, 1908. The following excerpts are from the minutes of the Council:

> "The cooperation with and the projected report of the Carnegie Foundation regarding medical colleges of the United States was discussed at length. Considerable objection was made to Chapter II, Part I. It was thought best to omit all of this part and to substitute a plea for an American standard of preliminary and medical education. ... It was considered wise to withhold publication of list of satisfactory colleges until the Carnegie Report comes out. This would shift some of the responsibility and that report would make the Council's report at a later date more effective."

Later that same afternoon, the Council met with Flexner and Pritchett.

> "At one o'clock an informal conference was held with President Pritchett and Mr. Abraham Flexner of the Carnegie Foundation. Mr. Pritchett had already expressed, by correspondence, the willingness of the Foundation to cooperate with the Council in investigating medical schools. He now explained that the Foundation was to investigate all the professions, law, medicine and theology. He had found no efforts being made by law to better the condition in legal education and had met with some slight opposition in the efforts he was making. He had then received the letters from the Council on Medical Education and expressed himself as most agreeably surprised not only at the efforts being made to correct conditions surrounding medical education but at the enormous amount of important data collected.
>
> "He agreed with the opinion previously expressed by the members of the Council that while the foundation would be guided very largely by the Council's investigations, to avoid the usual claims of partiality no more mention should be made in the report of the Council than

any other source of information. The report would therefore be, and have the weight of an independent report of a disinterested body, which would then be published far and wide. It would do much to develop public opinion."

Flexner had prepared an outline of his projected report as preparation for this meeting. A copy of the outline was found with the Flexner papers in the Library of Congress. In his original outline, Flexner argued that a uniform minimum of adequate medical instruction was "inadvisable and impossible". He argued that the facilities were not around at present to give everyone the most exacting type of education and that competent practitioners could be produced with less training than pure medical researchers. He argued that the diversity which marked the different areas of the United States could easily apply to medical education as well. In other words, Flexner initially argued that the current low and uneven level of medical education in the United States was a barrier to establishing a standard for future medical education and that it was advisable to have regional norms rather than a national one. The members of the Council on Medical Education objected to this section of the proposed report. They argued that an absolute minimum national standard was necessary or else the current situation would just be recreated. When the Flexner Report was finally published in 1910, it called for a uniform standard of medical education in the United States and Canada.

Shortly after this meeting, Flexner began the actual fieldwork for his study of medical education which entailed site visits to every one of the 155 medical schools in the United States and Canada. He began to visit the schools in January, 1909 in the company of Dr. N.P. Colwell, Secretary of the Council on Medical Education of the AMA. His pattern was to visit six or so schools and then return to New York to write up his notes. In general, he sought data on five points:

1 The entrance requirements—What were they and were they enforced?
2 The size and training of the faculty.
3 The sum available from endowment and fees for the support

of the institution and how it was allocated.
4 The quality and adequacy of the laboratories and the qualifications and training of the laboratory teachers.
5 The relations between the medical school and hospitals including the freedom of access to beds and freedom in the appointment by the school of the hospital physicians and surgeons.

In his autobiography, Flexner defended his cursory examination of each school by noting that Gates of the GEB used to remark: "You don't need to eat a whole sheep to know it's tainted" [1960: 78-9]. Flexner described one of his visits in the following way:

"In half an hour or less I could sample the credentials of students filed in the dean's office, ascertain the matriculation requirements (two years of high-school work, high-school graduation, two years of college work, or, finally, a college degree), and determine whether or not the standards, low or high, set forth in the school catalogue were being evaded or enforced. A few inquiries made clear whether the faculty was composed of local doctors, not already professors in some other local medical school, or the extent to which efforts had been made to obtain teachers properly trained elsewhere. A single question elicited the amount of income of a medical school, and a slight operation in mental arithmetic showed the approximate amount available for full-time teachers or for distribution as 'dividends' among the practising physicians who were 'professors'. A stroll through the laboratories disclosed the presence or absence of apparatus, museum specimens, library, and students; and a whiff told the inside story regarding the manner in which anatomy was cultivated. Finally, the situation as respects clinical facilities was readily clarified by a few questions, directed in succession—and separately—to the dean of the school, the professors of medicine, surgery, and obstetrics, and the hospital superintendent—questions which were designed to ascertain the extent to which the school enjoyed rights or merely courtesies in the hospitals named in the school catalogue. In the course of a few hours a reliable estimate could be made respecting the possibilities of teaching modern medicine in almost any of the 155 schools I visited in the United States and Canada." [1960: 79]

Flexner typed his reports in New York and then sent a copy

to the dean of the school with a request that any misstatements be corrected. Flexner noted:

> "I had the feeling during the whole time that the faculties were more than candid with me, because, though I endeavored to disabuse them of the idea, they were convinced that Mr. Carnegie, having once made a gift to a medical school in Atlanta, contemplated further activities of the same kind." [1960: 80]

I have found no evidence that such a gift was ever made by Carnegie. The fieldwork was completed in March, 1910 and the final version of the Flexner Report was released on June 11, 1910. The total cost of the Report was $14,000 (MacDonald 1956: 47). Pritchett sent a copy of the Report to Andrew Carnegie with the following comments:

> "I sent you on Saturday a copy of the report on Medical Education in the United States issued by the Foundation. The report has raised widespread interest in the medical profession and out of it, and you will doubtless see something of the mass of comment made upon it. It's the first thorough going effort to tell the truth about institutions which profess, in many cases, to stand on an altruistic basis, when as a matter of fact, they are in business ..." [Carnegie Papers, Library of Congress]

Throughout the course of the Report, Pritchett had developed a close rapport with Arthur Dean Bevan, Chairman of the Council on Medical Education. On November 4, 1909 Pritchett wrote to Bevan:

> "In all of this work of the examination of medical schools we have been hand in glove with you and your committee. In fact, we have only taken up the matter and gone on with the examination very much as you were doing, except that as an independent agency disconnected from actual practice, we may do certain things which you perhaps may not. When our report comes out it is going to be ammunition in your hands. It is desirable, therefore, to maintain in the meantime a position which does not intimate an immediate connection between our two efforts." [Carnegie Foundation Files]

Shortly after the publication of the Report (June 18, 1910), Pritchett again wrote to Bevan. He noted that there was not "more stone throwing than was to be expected". He called Bevan's attention to the "timidity on the part of the better medical men to stand by their guns in the matter of the report" and he wanted more public support from "men of stronger medical positions". He acknowledged that the criticism of the report as being "in a few places a little too sharp and has a somewhat dogmatic appearance" had "some weight". He also said:

> "I have been a little amused at the effort which has been made in a good many quarters to identify the Foundation in this matter with the so-called medical trust, which I understand to be mainly the American Medical Association and your Committee on Medical Education. Of course, this sort of cry does not disturb me at all." [Carnegie Foundation Files, June 18, 1910]

In reply, some months later, Bevan wrote:

> "You say that you are amused that the effort has been made to identify the foundation with the so-called 'Medical Trust'. I can only say that as a part of the American Medical Association that we feel very much flattered by such an association. I think that both the Foundation and the Medical Association can only be strengthened by attacks of this kind." [Carnegie Foundation Files, December 17, 1910]

The Flexner Report

Many people identify Bulletin Number Four of the Carnegie Foundation for the Advancement of Education, the *Flexner Report*, as a muckraking document that exposed the sorry state of medical education in the United States in the early twentieth century. But in actuality, the Report was far more than that. It was an attempt, much as Pritchett had wanted, to look at medical education through the eyes of a professional educator and to suggest a plan for the reformulation of medical education along more scientific lines.

If there is one argument that pervades the entire Report, it is that the number of physicians in the United States was far too high and that too many were being produced. Other countries had fewer and better doctors.

The Report began with a discussion of the history of medical

A System of Scientific Medicine

education in the United States. It includes a chapter discussing what the proper basis of medical education should be and another chapter discussing the actual basis of medical education. There follows four chapters on the suggested course of study and a chapter on the financial aspects of medical education. A plan for the reconstruction of medical education in the United States is set forth along with arguments about medical sects, state boards of licensure, postgraduate education, medical education for women, and medical education for blacks. The actual summary of the findings for each individual school follows in the second part of the book.

I will review some of the major arguments that Flexner used in Part I of the Report. These arguments reveal both the ideological framework of the Carnegie Foundation and the American Medical Association as well as the basis upon which medical education was reconstructed in the period after the Report. The major issues are: 1) "poor boy"; 2) need for college education; 3) pre-clinical (laboratory years); 4) clinical education and the hospital; 5) women and negro medical education; 6) plan for reorganization of medical education.

One of the conventional justifications for having medical school training last less than two years and of having minimal requirements for entrance into medical practice was so that the "poor boy" or economically disadvantaged individual could become a doctor. Flexner's critique of the "poor boy" argument not only set the tone for the Report, but was a major ideological argument. To begin his discussion of this issue, Flexner raised the question:

> "For whose sake is it permitted? [the lack of educational standards] Not really for the remote mountain districts of the south, for example, whence the 'yarb doctor', unschooled and unlicensed, can in no event be dislodged; nor yet for that twilight zone, on the hither edge of which so many low-grade doctors huddle that there is no decent living for those already there and no tempting prospect for anybody better: ostensibly, 'for the poor boy'. For his sake, the terms of entrance upon a medical career must be kept low and easy. We have no right, it is urged, to set up standards which will close the profession to 'poor boys'." [Flexner 1910: 42]

Abraham Flexner and the Flexner Report

Flexner addressed this argument by making six points:

1. No one has an inherent right to become a doctor because medicine is a social need not an individual obligation.
2. Medical education is not necessarily that expensive; therefore if poor boys would shop around, they could find a good medical education for the same price they pay for a bad one. Since thrift will be of the essence when poor boys become physicians, why not start early?
3. Poverty should not be an excuse for ignorance; therefore society should not allow inferior doctors just to remedy individual poverty.
4. It is wasteful to society to spend money on people who will not make good physicians when society could save money by training fewer but better doctors.
5. Poor boys don't go back to poor towns so there is no basis to the argument that if bad medical schools are closed down, the rural areas will be left without physicians.
6. It is in fact the very small and rural towns and areas that are in need of the best physicians, since they will have so much work to do; so poorly trained physicians should not be channeled to these areas.

Of all the changes that have ensued in medicine since the publication of the Flexner Report in 1910, the change in the class composition of the medical labor force has been the most significant. It is notable that Flexner did not recommend a scholarship program for worthy but needy youth seeking to become physicians. In general though, his recommendations are certainly consistent with other Progressive Era critiques of the quality of occupational candidates for advanced study.

Flexner recommended a high school diploma and two years of college level science as a minimum requirement for admission to medical school. He argued that students without this basis of training would be unable to utilize adequate laboratory facilities. He also noted that it would be difficult immediately to adopt this uniform standard and noted that for some time there would have to be three sets of standards: the high school and two years of college for most students; the higher standards for the better schools (e.g. Hopkins) and a special standard for the southern schools where the colleges tended to give the education that high schools did in other parts of the country.

Flexner recommended a four-year medical school curriculum in which the first two years would be totally consumed with the laboratory sciences. According to Flexner, students should take anatomy (including histology and embryology) and physiology (including biochemistry) in their first year and take pharmacology, pathology, bacteriology and physical diagnosis in their second year. Flexner noted that the physician must be a scientist first and must know and utilize the scientific method on an everyday basis. He stressed that teachers must do research on a continuing basis so that they could inspire the students.

The last two years of medical school were to be the clinical years and they were to be based in the hospital wards and dispensaries. The hospital, in Flexner's view, was a laboratory for scientific clinical investigation and observation, and the scientific method was just as important there as in the laboratory. Thus the professors of clinical specialties had to be scientists as well as practitioners. Moreover the medical school had to control the hospital so that the students' educational endeavors would not be bypassed. Ideally the hospital should have 200 to 300 beds continually filled so that students would not suffer a lack of clinical teaching material.

In an essay review of the Flexner Report, Chapman (1974:108) criticized Flexner for not seeming to understand that there was an art of medicine as well as a science. He noted that:

"His [Flexner's] language leaves little doubt that he held the massproduced 'family doctor' in low esteem and considered the ne plus ultra among physicians to be the highly scientific and sophisticated clinician moulded in the Hopkins environment or its equivalent. His words intensified a polarization within the medical profession that persists to this day between the specialist with five or more years of post-M.D. training, board certification, and, very often, full or parttime university faculty connections on the one hand, and the general practitioner, often with only one year of post-M.D. training and no university faculty connection on the other hand."

Flexner argued that the opportunities for coeducation in medicine were great and that therefore there was no need for medical schools specifically devoted to women. He recommended that all three schools for women be closed down. Yet, he also noted that "Now that women are freely admitted to the medical profession, it is clear that they show a decreasing inclination to enter it"(1910:178).

Flexner argued that there would always be a need for negro physicians even though some of the care of the negro would be provided by whites. His argument was largely that negroes needed their own physicians because negroes were a "potential source of infection and contagion" (1910:180). He recommended that the seven negro medical schools be reduced to two.

In his most ambitious section, he argued for the reconstruction of medical education along the themes noted in his report. He called for reducing the number of medical schools from 155 to 31, a number he felt would provide a sufficient quantity of physicians for the next thirty years. He based his arguments on the following premises: 1) the medical school should be a university department; 2) the medical school should be located in a large city so that access to clinical material (i.e. patients with varied ailments) would not be a problem; 3) there should only be one medical school per town or city; 4) the medical schools in each region should study regional problems. For example, in New Orleans the medical school should study tropical medicine and in Pittsburg the medical school should study occupational medicine.

In determining which schools should remain open, Flexner used what would be described today as a cost-effectiveness analysis. He looked at the various medical schools in a region and determined which ones had the greatest chance of becoming like his ideal and which ones would cost too much to reformulate. He argued for this reconstruction on the basis of rationality and economics but he also noted:

> "Society forbids a company of physicians to pour out upon the community a horde of ill-trained physicians. Their liberty is indeed clipped. As a result, however, more competent doctors are being trained

under the auspices of the state itself, the public health is improved; the physical well-being of the wage-worker is heightened; and a restriction put upon the liberty, so called, of a dozen doctors increases the effectual liberty of all other citizens. Has democracy, then, really suffered a set-back? Reorganization along rational lines involves the strengthening, not the weakening, of democratic principles, because it tends to provide the conditions upon which well-being and effectual liberty depend." [1910:155]

The second part of the Flexner Report is the better known of the two. It consists of Flexner's general comments regarding each state of the United States and the provinces of Canada along with a summary of what he found at each medical school in the state or province. The candor of the descriptions of the schools gave the Report its initial zest and was the major reason that the media covered the Report so extensively. To give a flavor of the Report, some examples, selected at random, are presented:

"The school occupies a few neglected rooms on the second floor of a fifty-foot frame building. Its so-called equipment is dirty and disorderly beyond description. Its outfit in anatomy consists of a small box of bones and the dried-up fragments of a single cadaver. A few bottles of reagents constitute the chemical laboratory. A cold and rusty incubator, a single microscope, and a few unlabeled wet specimens, etc., form the so-called 'equipment' for pathology and bacteriology." [p.190]

"Prominent among these [clinical facilities] is the so-called 'University Hospital', which may be cited as a typical instance of the misleading character of catalogue representations. The title itself is a misnomer; for the hospital is a university hospital not in the sense that large teaching advantages exist for the benefit of the university, but only in the sense that to the existing opportunities, restricted as they are, students from other schools are not admitted at all. The catalogue states that 'it contains one hundred beds, and its clinical advantages are used exclusively for the students of this college.' Not, however, the 'clinical advantages' of the 'one hundred beds', for 52 of them are private. Its 'clinical advantages' shrink on investigation to three weekly amphitheater clinics of slight pedagogic value and four ward clinics in obstetrics,—each of the latter attended by some 12 or 14 students in a ward containing 13 beds." [p.209]

Abraham Flexner and the Flexner Report

"Teaching staff: 45, 23 being full professors, 22 of other grade. No teacher devotes entire time to the school." [p.271]

" Entrance requirement: Less than a high school education." [p.291]

It was quotations like these that gave the local daily newspapers a reason for giving the Report wide exposure. These were also the quotations that have made people remember the Report. It is notable that while several threats of lawsuits for libel were made, none was actually carried out.

9
The Response to the Flexner Report

Upon its release in June 1910, the Flexner Report on Medical Education in the United States and Canada received a tremendous amount of press attention. The Carnegie Foundation printed 15,000 copies of the report for distribution at no charge. At the same time, Flexner summarized his report in *The Atlantic* and other magazines.

John Shaw Billings, the architect of the Johns Hopkins School of Medicine and one of the leading health statesmen of the period, wrote to Andrew Carnegie after reading the report to say:

"I feel impelled to tell you that the report on medical education in the United States and Canada, recently issued by Mr. Pritchett is in my opinion a very fine piece of work and one which I think will do good in the line of 'advancement of teaching'. When Johns Hopkins was being organized I investigated this matter and made recommendations, which, I think had some influence on the organization of that school. I therefore know something about the subject and Mr. Flexner's report appears to me to be a very accurate one. I hope that an equally good report will be made on the teaching of Law and Theology." [Carnegie Papers, June 14, 1910, Library of Congress]

To the newspapers of the day, the Flexner Report was banner headlines and front page news. Given the intense curiosity of the press for all things medical, the spiciness of the Report itself and

Response to the Flexner Report

the fact that it had examined and reviewed institutions across the entire North American continent made it marketable as news across the country. News of the Report was announced in the *Chicago Tribune*, the *Los Angeles Daily Times*, and the *New York Times*. It was also covered in such papers as the *Knoxville [Tennessee] Sentinel*, the *Omaha Bee*, and the *El Paso News*. Surely, this was exactly what the Council on Medical Education had desired when it said "it [the Report] would be published far and wide." Nevertheless the newspaper coverage while extensive and allowing for a great deal of editorial commentary, did not in itself have any serious impact on national medical policy. After all in a period of "yellow journalism", there were expositions like this one all the time. The furore over one would last until the next one was printed.

The international reaction was best typified by what was printed in the British journal *Nature*. Its report of September 15, 1910, coming three months after the publication, provided a less heated review.

"The Carnegie Foundation has a dual function, to provide pensions for the profession in the United States and Canada, and to 'encourage, uphold, and dignify the cause of higher education.' It is in connection with the latter that the trustees have undertaken a study of medical education in these countries. The report, prepared by Mr. Abraham Flexner, a trained chemist [sic], is in many respects a remarkable document, the publication of which, we are not surprised to hear, has caused a great sensation. There is no country in the world with medical schools at once so good and so bad as the United States. It would be hard to parallel in Europe conditions so favourable to the study of medicine at Harvard or the Johns Hopkins. On the other hand, a very large number of the medical schools are on a purely commercial basis, and offer an entirely inadequate education.... The condition of some of the commercial schools is scarcely conceivable, and Chicago is well called, in respect to medical education, the plague-spot of the United States. Englishmen will read with interest the report on the condition of medical education in Canada, and it is nice to hear that in point of construction and equipment the Toronto and Montreal laboratories are among the best on the continent. Praise is meted out to the medical school in the comparatively new city of Winnipeg. It is the purpose of the Foundation to proceed at once with a similar study of medical education in Germany, France and Great Britain, 'in order that those charged with the reconstruction of medical education in America may profit by the improvements in other countries.' We understand that Mr. Flexner will be in this country early in October to pursue his work. The report cannot but be most helpful. It is thoroughly well done; perhaps the only legitimate criticism is an insufficient appreciation by its author of the extraordinary progress which higher medical education has made in the United States in the past twenty-five years." [*Nature*, September 15, 1910, p.333]

The American medical journals, however, having more at stake in the content of the the Flexner Report and being somewhat more in touch with the issues, had at best mixed reactions and, for the most part, even the more 'enlightened' medical journals were somewhat cool to the Report in their reviews. The *Journal of the American Medical Association* (*JAMA*), for example, agreed with everything the Report had to say. Not acknowledging any prior collaborative efforts between the American Medical Association (AMA) and the Carnegie Foundation, the *Journal* editorial included the following passage which commented on the presumed impartiality of the research:

> "This report is evidently the result of an enormous amount of painstaking work and is worthy of the most careful study. Coming from an agency outside and independent of the medical profession, it is sure to have a most profound influence on medical education in general, and claims of partiality or prejudice cannot be made against it." [June, 1910:1949]

Nevertheless, the entire two-page editorial is not as exuberant in its praise of the Report as might be expected given the prior understanding between the AMA and the Carnegie Foundation. It may well be that the AMA was somewhat piqued at not being mentioned at all in the report (as per the arrangement worked out in advance). Several weeks later, on July 23, 1910 the *JAMA* had another comment on the Report, this being a short roundup of other press comments. It cited two or three newspaper articles which agreed with the recommendations of the Report. In acknowledging the criticisms the Report received, the journal read: "Although there may be statements of detail which might be

Response to the Flexner Report

criticized in the Foundation's report, generally speaking the statements made are recognized as the truth by those who are in a position to judge" (p.318).

Other journals of the day were more critical. The *Medical Record*, a weekly medical journal which covered all facets of medicine and was supportive of scientific medicine, was rather pointed in its editorial remarks:

"The report professes to be based on a thorough and most painstaking personal investigation of every medical school of this country and Canada, made by Mr. Abraham Flexner, a professional critic of educators, student of systems of education. In order to correct every current misconception, we may say, in parenthesis, that this is not Dr. Simon Flexner of the Rockefeller Institute, but his brother. The doctor has trouble of his own with the antis of various ilks, and should not lose professional support through being made to answer for the sins of his brother. Neither, may we add, should the brother be judged by the essay which the president of the Foundation [Pritchett] contributes by way of introduction to the report. . . . What the writer does not seem to have discovered is that all these schools, with the exception of a very small and practically negligible number, are in the process of betterment, and that several associations of medical men and medical educators are working constantly to encourage and force the poorer schools to raise their standards and improve their teaching methods. When one realizes what the best of medical schools were twenty-five or thirty years ago, and what tremendous progress has been made during the past twenty, and especially the past ten years, and when one remembers that all this uplift has come from within, without the help of any outside 'Foundation' the work of Mr. Flexner seems somewhat a waste of effort and a needless expenditure of Mr. Carnegie's hard-earned money. . . . The writers of the Bulletin are unfair in that they ignore what has already been accomplished and are silent as to agencies at work in raising the standards of medical education. Whether this omission of a fact which, if properly presented, would prove the work of the foundation to have been one of supererogation, was intentional or whether it is only evidence of a superficial and one-sided investigation, we do not know." [June 25, 1910:1097]

The *New York State Journal of Medicine* was also critical of the Report, in part for the same reasons and in part for more political reasons:

"If it is unwise for the State, the legally constituted guardian of the liberties of the people, the grantor of the charters of all corporate bodies, whether of commerce or institution, to dictate the policies and methods of its own universities, what shall we say concerning a foundation itself the creature of the state which arrogates to itself powers not possessed by the State? An oligarchy within a republic is an anomaly. It is not the less anomalous because its intentions are good if its methods are such as to threaten the freedom of educational institutions ... [This section included a long critique of the Carnegie rules for pensions etc.] ... The development of such an institution in our midst is abnormal and unhealthy. An oligarchy has no place in a democracy, nor should the mere possession of or access to great wealth by the means of engrafting in our midst a sort of supreme educational council, self-perpetuating, responsible to no one — in fact, an education oligarchy with the vast inertia of an immense fortune behind it. Trade and commerce have for years been suffering from the dictation of powerful interests which have well nigh outgrown control both of courts and legislatures. ... What newspaper in the country would have dared publish on its own initiative, such a wholesale and intemperate criticism of the medical schools of the country as was contained in Bulletin No. IV ? The fear of the laws against libel would have restrained them. When they did comment on Bulletin No. IV, it was always with the careful use of quotation marks. ... Nowhere in the Bulletin has any credit been given to the medical profession for the earnest and sincere efforts which it has been making this quarter of a century to improve the status of medical education. Have we no laws in every State of the Union, laws compelling the graduates of every school to submit to a severe state examination before admission to practice? Who originated these laws? Was it a layman, a teacher of secondary schools? These reforms were initiated before the critic of the Bulletin was out of short clothes, in the State of New York by the Medical Society of the State of New York and have extended throughout the United States. We have not sought improvement by fiat and imperial edict. We have not sought to wipe out institutions with the stroke of a pen. We have said to the various medical schools through the voice of our State Board of Examiners 'Mend your ways or your students will get no license.' More than that the American Medical Association established some years ago a Council on Medical Education whose methods have been moderate but persuasive. Time mends all things. Fiat education is just as bad as fiat money—and as legal. If the methods which the Carnegie Foundation tends to employ in the future may be judged by its recent pronunciamento and the changes which its board of trustees have recently demanded, its benefits are little to be desired by self-respecting men or institutions." [November, 1910: 483-84]

A last comment is worth citing. This appeared under the heading 'Medical Socialism' in the *Medical Notes and Queries*, a Pennsylvania medical journal for practitioners:

"Among the many forces crowding and driving our land into socialism, medicine may well be considered as the most powerful, as it was also the earliest in the field. It had long since, with hospitals and dispensaries, begun to give the object lessons that the world requires. Already in its boards of health and in its health legislation, in the quarantines that it establishes, and in its demand for the registration of diseases it exhibits the tyranny of the masses over the individual, and now it has a new evangelist.... For the men who raise standards and condemn institutions as below par are not willing to step down and do the active work of the profession, nor should they; but who, when the despised four-fifths are eliminated, will do it? Only by rearranging matters, by making medical districts of the whole land, on the Swiss plan; by allotting to each its medical officer or officers, and by casting adrift the unlucky four-fifths. In short this new institute, these few men, are already assuming the right to manage the profession, to overthrow its traditions and to rebuild it on Socialistic lines." [June, 1910: 123-25]

With the success of the Report assured by the press attention it received, Flexner was rewarded with a raise in salary to $5,000 per year. He was also given his next assignment, which was to write a report on European medical education. This was a subject that had arisen earlier and to which the Carnegie Foundation and Pritchett had agreed. Flexner was to be dispatched to Germany, England and France to study their systems of medical education. All agreed it should have been done first, however the essence of the second report was expected to confirm that medical education in the United States was on the right track. Flexner left for Europe in the summer of 1910 and returned sometime during 1911. The report was published in 1912 as Bulletin Number Six of the Carnegie Foundation and titled *Medical Education in Europe*.

A System of Scientific Medicine

With respect to the future development of the American medical care system, a very important event happened in 1911 at a meeting among Flexner and Gates, the Chairman of the General Education Board, and other Rockefeller philanthropies. In medical folklore, the meeting between Flexner and Gates seems to have taken on mythological stature but interestingly the only account of it was Flexner's. The sum and substance of the discussion between the men, as reported by Flexner were as follows:

> "I have read your 'Bulletin Number Four' from beginning to end. It is not only a criticism; it is also a program. I replied, It was intended, Mr. Gates, to be both, for you will remember that it contains two maps: one showing the location and number of medical schools in America today; the other showing what, in my judgement, would suffice if medical schools were properly endowed and conducted. What would you do, asked Mr. Gates, if you had a million dollars with which to make a start in the work of reorganizing medical education? Without a moment's hesitation, I replied, I should give it to Dr. Welch. Why? With an endowment of four hundred thousand dollars, I answered, Dr. Welch has created, in so far as it goes, the one ideal medical school in America. Think what he might do if he had a million more. Already the work Dr. Welch and his associates have done in Baltimore is having its effect in reorganizing the personnel of medical schools elsewhere, and we must not forget that but for Johns Hopkins Medical School there would be no Rockefeller Institute for Medical Research in New York today. Would Pritchett release you long enough to go to Baltimore to make a detailed study of the situation and report to me? I think he would, I replied. Ask him, and if he agrees, go. Thereupon the luncheon terminated. Dr. Pritchett was extremely happy to realize that 'Bulletin Number Four' might have practical consequences of importance, and he made it possible for me to spend a period of about three weeks in Baltimore." [1960: 109–10]

As noted above, the source of much of this information was Flexner himself, and virtually all subsequent renderings of this account are based on Flexner's version. Gates, for example, in his autobiography, did not mention this luncheon and explained this assignment he gave to Flexner as his attempt to help out Dr. Welch and Johns Hopkins. It should be noted that Welch, Simon Flexner and others on the staff of the Rockefeller Institute were faculty at Hopkins and Welch and Simon Flexner had become the most important advisors to Gates on medical matters. Gates's version of the story in his autobiography follows:

> "My attention had been drawn to Johns Hopkins, of course, by Dr. Osler's book and Mr. Rockefeller had given many years before this some Four Hundred Thousand Dollars to Johns Hopkins Medical School to make good its losses in the great Baltimore fire [1904]. It was in 1911, I think, that Dr. Welch sought from Mr. Rockefeller a new and considerable gift for Johns Hopkins Medical School. After conference with my associates in Mr. Rockefeller's office, we promised to support Dr. Welch, on condition that the clinical chair at Hopkins be placed on a full-time basis. Dr. Welch himself had long approved the idea. Dr. [Simon] Flexner warmly supported it, and both began a quiet advocacy of 'Full Time' among the trustees and faculty of Hopkins. Months and even years passed. Dr. Abraham Flexner was finally sent to Hopkins to make a complete study of costs and other elements of the situation." [1977: 232]

In the oral history archives at Columbia University, there is a transcript of an interview with Abraham Flexner conducted when he was eighty-eight years old (December, 1954). The account of the meeting presented in that interview is so divergent from other historical records, that one must assume that Flexner had confused his dates and facts by that time. Nevertheless, although the accuracy of this version is highly suspect, it is presented here in the interests of completeness:

> "Then later when I got to making the survey for the Carnegie Foundation in 1910 I went down and spent three or four weeks at the [Johns Hopkins] hospital mainly with Dr. Welch. Subsequent to that Mr. Frederick T. Gates once asked me, 'If you had a million dollars what would you do with it?' I said, 'I'd give it to Dr. Welch.' 'All of it?' 'Yes.' 'Why?' 'Well, I said, he's been running Hopkins on an endowment of $500,000, which means that it's run really on tuition, and the school is twice as large as it ought to be. If he had a million dollars perhaps he could cut the school down.' So he said, 'Would Henry Pritchett let you go and make a study for me?' I said, 'Yes, I'm sure he would.' So I went back to Baltimore and spent a month. At the end of the month I made a report for Mr. Gates, in the course of which I said, 'You can't do anything with a million dollars. It would

take a million and a half. With a million and a half they could cut the school down and institute full time, in the main, clinical chairs.'
... [Interviewer: Gates accepted your report without any question and he spoke to Mr. Rockefeller about it?] Oh yes. That led Mr. Gates to ask me to lunch one day. He said, 'I've been reading your report. It's not only a criticism. It's a program.' I said, 'Mr. Gates, that's what it was meant to be. There are two maps in it—one showing the location of every medical school in the United States and Canada, 155 of them; the other showing what, in my judgement, the country needs.' He said, 'How much would it cost to convert the first map into the second?' I said, 'It might cost a billion dollars.' Mr. Gates said, 'All right, we've got the money. Come down here and we'll give it to you.' I said, 'You can't do it that way, Mr. Gates. The country won't stand for Mr. Rockefeller doing it alone.' He said, 'Well how much will the country stand?' 'Well,' I said, 'I think if you gave $50 million, (I don't know why I settled on $50 million) I think I could raise the rest.' He said, 'All right. Come down here and we'll give you $50 million.' Then I said, 'I must first approach Mr. Carnegie, the person who financed this study.' Mr. Gates said, 'That's only fair.' So I told Mr. Pritchett and the next day we went up to see Mr. Carnegie, and I told him. He said, 'I don't believe Mr. Gates will do it.' Why not? 'You've proved medical teaching is a business and I won't endow anybody's business.' I said, 'If you endow it, Mr. Carnegie, it won't be a business.' He said, 'I don't think you can change these men.' I said, 'I don't propose to change them. I propose to get rid of them.' He couldn't see it, and I left [presumably the Carnegie Foundation]. He said, 'I'll get you back.' I said, 'No you won't.' " [Flexner 1959:17-20]

The next chapter will relate what happened at Johns Hopkins over the next several years, a story compiled from a multitude of sources that outlines the initial changes in medical education that were implemented under the aegis of the Rockefeller GEB over the next twenty years. These developments completely changed the face of American medicine. It is important to note that though the changes that were brought about in medical education were done under the stewardship of Abraham Flexner, the actual changes were, in several important respects, far different from what had been recommended in the original Flexner Report of 1910. This has proven to be an immense stumbling block for historians of medical education as they try to identify the reasons why contemporary medical education does not resemble the ideals laid out in the famous Bulletin Number Four of 1910. What the following chapter will show is that Flexner was hired to implement reforms in which he may have come to believe but reforms that he did not think were critical to his original analysis of medical education in the United States and Canada. That Flexner presided over the reforms and has presided over the writing of the history only serves to further deflect the fact that the full-time plan was a creation of the foundations, for good or bad, rather than a creation by Flexner. At this point in time, seventy-five years after the publication of the Flexner Report, it is still necessary to underscore this fundamental, but largely unknown, historical point.

10
Foundations and Medical Education — 1910–35

The previous chapter explored the role of the large philanthropic foundations in giving impetus and financial support to the growing scientific medicine movement in America from the 1890s to the publication of the Flexner Report in 1910. While medical education was not totally neglected, it is apparent that the main thrust of philanthropic largesse rested in the establishment of facilities conducive to medical research.

The foundations were not yet prepared to directly support medical education, as the case of the McGill Medical School reveals, though they were aware of the need for improvement. The growing movement of medical self-reform and the public impact of the Flexner Report set the stage for generous foundation support for medical education. While the large foundations never abandoned their extensive financial support of basic research, they clearly shifted the emphasis of their giving toward medical education. It is notable though that the medical education which was supported by foundation money always emphasized medical research as an integral component of professional preparation. The period from the 1890s to 1910 can be viewed as the era of foundation support for medical research, thus establishing the groundwork for scientific medicine. The period from 1910 to 1935 was an era of foundation support for medical education. There is nothing absolute about those dates, although they do allow for the demarcation of the shifting emphasis of philanthropic support. In terms of medicine and medical care, the most significant development that occurred during this later period was the emergence of the hospital as a focal point of the medical care system.

The Rockefeller-endowed GEB was the major private supporter of scientific medicine in the United States between 1910 and 1935. Rockefeller philanthropies were responsible for 90–95 per cent of all foundation money going into medicine at this time and therefore any analysis of this period must concern itself primarily with the Rockefeller philanthropies. Because of the centrality of private philanthropic foundations to the development of the medical care system, it is important to consider the changes that were occurring within the foundations and within American society as the foundations became better known institutions and as the dangers of large sums of money in private control became the focus of national debate.

Foundations had typically been met with distrust and, in some cases, outright hostility on the part of the public. Their small size and limited scope, as well as their interest in groups and people who were at the margins of society (e.g. southern blacks, southern farmers, rural peoples, etc.), tended to shield the foundations from direct criticism. Very few people knew what foundations were doing and therefore no one really cared. As foundations began to shift their objectives toward more mainstream activities and began to direct their attention toward more powerful elements of society, the degree of public outcry began to increase. This change in public perception can be seen in the difference in ease of obtaining a congressional charter by two Rockefeller philanthropies.

In 1903, the GEB was granted a charter by the Congress of the United States. Senator Nelson Aldrich of Rhode Island, the father-in-law of Rockefeller, Jr., single-handedly pushed the charter bill through Congress with little dissent. In 1911, attempts were made to obtain a congressional charter for the Rockefeller Foundation. After two years of heavily publicized fighting and attempts at compromise the Foundation was not given a charter. This delay and eventual denial was attributed to its inability to agree to several stipulations that the Congress wanted to attach to a charter.

A System of Scientific Medicine

Among the compromises discussed were: 1) having the President, Vice President, Chief Justice of the Supreme Court, Speaker of the House of Representatives, and the Presidents of Johns Hopkins, Harvard, Yale, Columbia and University of Chicago choose future trustees of the Foundation; 2) allowing no further build-up of principal; 3) allowing Congress to make changes in the charter at congressional request. The Foundation was instead inconspicuously given a charter by New York State in 1913 (Fosdick 1952:17-20).

A variety of factors led to this change in reception for private philanthropic foundations. The publication of Ida Tarbell's *History of the Standard Oil Company*, after its earlier serialization in *McCall's* magazine was a major source of public disaffection with the Rockefellers. The tale of Rockefeller, Sr.'s ruthless quest for money and the vivid stories of small farmers and oil explorers driven to poverty by Rockefeller's tawdry tactics did little to endear the man to the public and led people to be suspicious of any sign of benevolence. The 1905 "tainted money" scandal in which a Congregational minister refused a Rockefeller donation because any money that came from Rockefeller had to be tainted with the blood that was shed for him to get it, also led to a vast public debate on whether social good could come from money whose origin was suspect. The 1907 court decision which fined the Standard Oil Company $29 million for restraint of trade, known popularly as the Landis decision, also contributed to the public antipathy toward "robber barons" and the means they used to acquire their wealth (Latham 1949).

Many people also had reason to suspect that the reason for the desire for congressional approval of the Rockefeller Foundation had much to do with the dissolution suit then pending against the Standard Oil Company and the more frequent discussions about a national income tax then pending in Congress. These were all criticisms of the founder and the origin of the money rather than criticisms of foundations in general or of their projects. The Rockefeller Sanitary Commission, then working on the eradication of hookworm throughout the South, at first met with wide criticism which was eventually muted due to the public acceptance of and appreciation for the campaign. The Rockefeller

Institute continued to receive favorable press as its discoveries and accomplishments received widespread attention and even the Carnegie Foundation which sponsored the Flexner Report met with general popular approval.

Yet, particularly in the next decade (1910-20), the public acceptance of philanthropic foundations, as well as foundation benefactors, began to change noticeably. A number of events linked foundations closely to their benefactors, in a manner which did not reflect well on the foundations. Moreover, much criticism was directed toward foundations from the groups receiving critical attention from the projects of the foundations. These were far more powerful groups within society than those with whom the foundations had dealt previously. An interesting phenomenon occurred—the agencies, institutions or organizations which the foundations first empowered through generous grants came to resent the continued intervention of the foundations in their activities.

A clear example of this resentment can be seen in the struggle of public school teachers through their professional organization, the National Educational Association (NEA), against the philanthropic foundations who were responsible for the very schools in which they taught and their jobs. Whatever professional power and prestige public school teachers enjoyed, came as a result of foundation gifts and benefactions that built new schools and upgraded the standards for teachers. In July, 1914, the NEA adopted the following resolution:

> "We view with alarm the activity of the Carnegie and Rockefeller Foundations, agencies not in any way responsible to the people, in their efforts to control the policies of our State educational institutions, to fashion after their conception and to standardize our courses of study, and to surround the institutions with conditions which menace true academic freedom and defeat the primary purpose of democracy as heretofore preserved and inviolable in our common schools, normal schools and universities." [Tentative draft reply to resolution of NEA, Rockefeller Foundation Archives]

While this resolution was viewed by the officers of the GEB as a 'faint roar in the distance after the somewhat violent thunderstorm at Washington' (presumably the struggle over the Rockefeller Foundation charter), and really directed against the Carnegie Foundation but that "they desire to lump us all together for fear that they might be called upon for a bill of particulars", the officers felt they had to respond (A. Flexner to W. Buttrick, July 15, 1914, Rockefeller Foundation Archives). The GEB issued a blanket denial of wrongdoing in any sense but also agreed to publish an annual report to keep the public informed as to what the foundation was doing.

Similarly, the universities which were the primary recipients of foundation grants were encouraged by the foundations to organize active, financially committed alumni and community constituencies as additional sources of revenue. As these groups formed, they began to resist what they perceived as foundation meddling in their affairs, and the institutions became demonstrably less dependent on the foundations for their financial viability (Curti and Nash 1965:134-35).

The incident which did the most to link foundations to the actions of their benefactors was the congressional investigation into labor violence held in 1915 (Commission on Industrial Relations 1916). The immediate cause for this investigation was the Ludlow Massacre of 1914, the willful and brutal murder of workers and their families in Ludlow, Colorado by a company controlled by the Rockefeller family and whose stock was held by the Rockefeller philanthropies (Horowitz and Collier 1975).

The Commission on Industrial Relations, chaired by Senator Frank Walsh, held hearings on the role of philanthropic foundations, as holders of large blocks of corporate stock, in perpetuating or alleviating labor violence. The Commission sought to answer questions regarding the role of the stockholder, (including the foundations) in corporate affairs. The pursuit of this inquiry involved the formal questioning of Andrew Carnegie, J.P. Morgan, Rockefeller, Sr., and Rockefeller, Jr., the latter of whom was questioned on three separate occasions by the Commission and eventually was found to have perjured himself. He had maintained that he had no role in the Colorado strike, but letters were introduced into testimony which showed that he had given his approval to the actions of the management of the company during the strike (Lanksford 1964).

Vast public outcry against philanthropic foundations resulted from these inquiries and the foundations themselves retreated from some of their more ambitious projects as a result. The next few years saw the large foundations engage in relatively benign activities such as war relief, until the public pressure abated (Fosdick 1952:27-9).

The growth and upgrading of the hospital

The most obvious change in medicine and medical care in the twentieth century was the newly found importance of the hospital. During the nineteenth century, the hospital in both Europe and America was used mostly by paupers and considered to be an almshouse or a deathhouse (Abel-Smith 1964).

In Britain, this role had been fostered by the Poor Laws. In 1861, only 14 out of 10,414 inpatients of hospitals were considered to be "persons of Rank or Property" (Freymann 1974). The introduction of anesthesia twenty years before the introduction of aseptic technique in surgery increased the death rates directly attributable to the hospital but did not serve to change the basic pattern of usage. The situation began to change when the British Medical Practice Act of 1858 declared large numbers of healers to be unqualified and forced the largely working class patients of these practitioners into the hospitals to receive their medical care (Turshen 1975:103).

In America, the situation was not much different. Public hospitals were set up in the larger cities during the first half of the nineteenth century as repositories for victims of infectious disease epidemics. As in Europe, this care was funded primarily through religious or civic philanthropy. For example, when Johns Hopkins, in his will, bequeathed a hospital along with a university, he stipulated that provision be made for paying patients although he noted that these could only be strangers to the community or people who had no relatives or friends to care for them in their sickness (Freymann 1974:66-7).

Toward the end of the nineteenth century and the beginning of the twentieth century, advances in technology led to a change in the function of the hospital. The introduction of X-ray machines in 1897 and the clinical laboratory in 1901 along with such developments as electric lighting, elevators and improved ventilation systems made the hospital more effective therapeutically as well as more comfortable. The increasing success of surgery practiced under antiseptic technique and the resultant decline of nosocomial infections (hospitalism) began to give the hospital a therapeutic mission, whereas previously it had served a largely domiciliary function. The increasing utility of the hospital spurred the growth of pay wards, which also served to offset some of the costs of the new technology that hospitals were adding. In 1895, speaking to an audience of the Boston social elite, Edward Everett Hale said:

> "One of the lessons of the Civil War of the utmost importance was that it taught us about hospitals. Some people do not believe it now but they will come to it before the twentieth century is over, that it is a great deal better to be sick in hospitals than to be sick in a house only half equipped for the purpose." [Freymann 1974:67]

By the first years of the twentieth century, the hospital had assumed a dual role. It still continued its historic function of care for the indigent but now added the new mission of rehabilitative haven for the wealthy. The Johns Hopkins Hospital, by gathering the best clinicians of the era (e.g. Osler, Kelly, Halstead, etc.) was in the vanguard of this movement. While there is only anecdotal evidence to support this conclusion, the number of letters contained in the archives of the Rockefeller philanthropies written on Johns Hopkins Hospital stationery suggests that the Trustees of the Foundation frequently used the facility for their medical care. By 1910, however, with the opening of the Hospital of the Rockefeller Institute in New York City, the use of Johns Hopkins in Baltimore declined.

By 1910, the new pattern of upper class usage of hospitals had been firmly established. Despite this change, only a small portion of people in the United States ever used a hospital—the very poor and the very rich. Even in 1912, according to an editorial in *Modern Hospital* magazine, only 13 per cent of the sick were treated in the hospital; the other 87 per cent being cared for at home (Reverby 1975: 8). By 1930 though, the hospital was clearly the center of the medical care delivery system. How did the hospital achieve such a dramatic shift in utilization in such a short period of time?

While the technological, scientific and comforting aspects of the hospital all contributed to its popularity, these were not the sole reasons for it. They do not explain why the hospital, rather than the physician's office, clinic, or other setting, became the focal point of medical care delivery. The importance of the hospital to the projects that were funded by philanthropic foundations was central to the increased utilization and therefore a brief discussion of the hospital is warranted and necessary.

Several basic economic reasons which promoted the expansion of the hospital were delineated in some of the medical journals of the era:

> "They [community hospitals] enable large employers of labor to pay smaller wages because the community, through its hospitals, takes the burden of the working man's illness." [Post 1908: 823]

and,

> "The manual tradesman at the moderate wage may have as prompt, effective, skillful, and even luxurious medical and surgical services as the bloated bondholder or the munificently remunerated professional man.... At the same time it [the hospital] is cheap. The house may be smaller if the births, sicknesses and surgical operations are provided for in the hospital. The wages may therefore be reduced, and yet the standard of life remain the same or even raised. From an economic point of view the hospital is a success. It is ready, quick and cheap. It is economy, therefore, for the employing class to build many hospitals at the expense of a few million rather than pay the wages necessary to keep their employees in equal decency in their confinements, sicknesses and surgical operations at home. Whether these hospitals are built as railway hospitals, as eleemosynary adjuncts of religious societies or as monuments of national or racial pride, matters not either to the exploiting capitalist or to the suffering patient. The result is the same, a diminution of waste, an economic gain and an increase in the technical efficiency, and a gradual rise in the standard of life." [Holmes 1906: 318-19]

A System of Scientific Medicine

and,

> "I venture to say that no town of 20,000 people can afford to be without its hospital for the sake of its own citizens, utterly irrespective of the good it does to the poor, who are treated in its wards. It must be established in the interest of the *well-to-do citizens* and their families so that they may secure better equipped doctors for themselves as well as for the patients in their hospitals. Self-interest, therefore, will compel every community to establish its hospital even if charitable motives had no influence." [Post 1908: 825, emphasis in original]

The hospital can be considered the analogue to the industrial factory. Just as the factory made it possible to eliminate marginal producers, the hospital made it possible to marginalize office-based practitioners. That hospitals can be considered as medical factories is more than just rhetorical flourish. An article appeared in *Modern Hospital* in 1916, entitled "The Modern Hospital as a Health Factory". The author argued that the hospital should be viewed not so much as a "collection of individually sick persons," but rather as "a health manufacturing plant ... which specializes in the conversion of the non-producing and wealth absorbing sick men and women into wealth producing citizens." (Reverby 1975: 17).

While it is possible to stretch the analogy too far, a comparison of the development of the hospital and the development of the factory is of interest. As Stephen Marglin demonstrated in his "What Do Bosses Do?", the factory did not emerge because it was a superior mechanism of production from an economic standpoint (Marglin 1974). It was, in fact, inferior to the cottage industry system on a cost basis. Its *raison d'être* revolved around the fact that it allowed for the capitalist to enter the production process and ensure discipline—on both workers and product. Similarly, the hospital allowed for the rigorous supervision of health workers and perhaps more important allowed for the standardization of illness and the illness experience. While most industries of the time had been or were undergoing de-skilling (that is—the replacement of skilled labor by machinery), the industrial system had created the need for a trained workforce which was always on the job (Stone 1974). While workers were typically fired or replaced when they got ill, the process was inefficient and costly and grew increasingly dysfunctional as the training levels of new employees increased. The hospital allowed the capitalist to impose discipline on the health habits of workers and to standardize both the illness and the treatment. This tendency to improve the economic efficiency of the hospital was best typified by such early standardization regimens as Codman's End-Product system which attempted to standardize surgical practice through quality control measures (Codman 1913). One could postulate that the real improvement of the hospital over the doctor's office or the clinic was in the standardization of diagnosis and treatment particularly in an era when large numbers of medical sects still existed and when physicians were trained in very different backgrounds and techniques. Moreover, the hospital served to legitimize much industrially induced pathology by acting as a repair shop.

As increasing numbers of the populace were drawn into the hospital and began to utilize it for their medical care, the system of medicine which became institutionalized in the public mind was a clinical system totally removed from the social realities outside the hospital walls. Clinicians, now permanently ensconced within the hospital, could only see disease as it presented itself from the hospital bed. The etiology of disease and the social factors that mediated, influenced, or caused it were excluded from what Foucault (1974) has called the clinical "gaze". The physician working inside the hospital had a distorted view of the actual extent and nature of the morbidity and mortality outside this clinical setting.

The hospital tended to replicate and hence reinforce the social relations of the factory. The hospital was characterized by a detailed division of labor and an elaborate hierarchy. Through its use of medical technology and equipment, the hospital tended to promote the emerging commodity form of medicine.

It can be argued, then, that the growth and increasing centrality of the hospital was mandated by the necessities of the political economy of the country. The trend toward the increased utilization of the hospital was abetted by two movements of the day—the drive for a compulsory national health insurance and the philanthropic foundation sponsored full-time clinical plan.

A System of Scientific Medicine

The American Association for Labor Legislation (AALL), a corporate research and policy group funded primarily by the wealthiest capitalists (Rockefeller, Morgan, Gary, Astor, and the Milbank, Carnegie and Russell Sage Foundations), was established in 1906. The AALL was active in promoting and lobbying for Workman's Compensation, industrial accident, and disease prevention, etc. It also attempted to establish a compulsory national health insurance system in the United States that operated at the state level (Domhoff 1970:170–79) Several members of the American Medical Association (AMA) hierarchy were active in the AALL and the journal of the AMA used its editorial pages to promote the idea of health insurance (Rayack 1967). Because the hierarchy of the AMA at this time consisted mostly of scientists and hence these people were based in hospitals, a health insurance scheme would have had little effect on them. Assured payment for hospital care would have in fact increased their income at the expense of office-based practitioners.

While the plan for national health insurance was being formulated in 1915 and 1916, it received much support within the ranks of the AMA. Since it offered health insurance only to industrial workers and to no one else, much like the European and British social insurance systems of the time, it was supported by large industrialists but opposed by a coalition made up of office-based physicians, insurance companies, and the National Association of Manufacturers, the trade organization of small businesses. While compulsory national health insurance did not win passage at that time (and still has not in the United States), the movement further focused attention on the hospital as the new center of medical care delivery.

The second movement was the full-time clinical plan that was supported primarily by the GEB. The story of the foundations' attempt to implement the full-time plan will be discussed in the following chapter.

11
The Full-time Plan

As noted earlier, Abraham Flexner was commissioned by Gates of the GEB to make a site visit at the Johns Hopkins Medical School and to report back to Gates. Flexner visited Baltimore either in February or early March, 1911. According to the account given in his autobiography, Flexner proposed that $1½ million be given to the Medical School in order to enable the reorganization of the medical, surgical, obstetrical, and pediatric clinics on a full-time basis (Flexner 1960: 112). Before going further into this story, it is necessary to give some background on the full-time plan, what it was and why Flexner should have recommended it when not a word about such a system of medical care was mentioned in the Flexner Report of 1910.

In essence, the full-time plan meant that professors of clinical medicine and clinical medical specialties in medical schools would be paid fixed salaries and their entire income would be derived from teaching and research. Any money that might be received from private practice or consulting work, if there were any such monies, would be collected by the Medical School and deposited in its treasury. This meant that the clinical faculty of the medical schools would be in the same position as the laboratory faculty; they would receive a salary and not be permitted to make any outside income. A modified version of this plan still dominates the teaching of clinical medicine in the United States today, known as the geographic full-time system.

A System of Scientific Medicine

Before elaborating on the details of the development of the full-time plan and the reasons the foundations became involved in it, some historical perspective on the development of teaching clinical medicine might be useful.

Before the advent of foundation support, medical schools tended to be parochial in their choice of faculty. Teaching faculty were generally local physicians who sought to earn additional income through teaching fees. Those who had a good reputation and a student following could generally earn additional consulting money from former students who would rely on their professors' expertise for difficult cases. In many cases faculty appointments were the result of nepotism and primogeniture. This approach to faculty appointments in medical education tended to impede the introduction of scientific methods and research into medicine in the United States (Rothstein 1972). As the Flexners note in their biography of William Welch:

> "Except at Hopkins, the professors who expounded actual methods of treating patients were still, as all American medical teachers had once been, selected from among the leading local practitioners; The Harvard Medical School, for instance, failed to call a clinical professor from the outside until 1912. Even the minor clinical posts were held by local doctors who often retained their appointments for most of their lives, in sharp contrast to the assistants or assistant professors in laboratory departments, who were young men appointed for a short term and expected to improve scientifically so that they could be advanced or to be called elsewhere. ... There was no way for a young man to get a clinical position through the whole-hearted pursuit of the scientific side of medicine." [Flexner and Flexner 1966: 298]

In addition, while laboratory scientists were paid extremely low salaries (the price one paid for being a scientist), the clinical faculty were often quite wealthy due to private practices and consultant work (Brown 1979: 158-64). This inequitable financial situation understandably generated some resentment from the laboratory scientists toward their wealthier brethren on the clinical side. It should be noted that until the turn of the century, this was not a major issue since few medical schools had any full-time laboratory staff at all. Before the Flexner Report, only anatomy was taught on a regular basis and that generally by a local surgeon on a part-time basis. As American students returned from German universities and research laboratories, having studied bacteriology and other new bio-medical sciences, they began to seek positions in American medical schools (Bonner 1963:107–37). The encouragement of research in medicine by the Rockefeller philanthropies in particular enabled many of these scientists to find jobs at medical schools; but even a casual reading of the Flexner Report reveals that the majority of medical schools did not have laboratories at all, let alone full-time scientific staffs (Flexner 1910). As American medicine began to develop and as an increasing number of medical schools began to build full-time laboratory and research departments, the plaint of the scientists became more audible.

The basic idea for the full-time plan originated in the German physiology laboratories of Carl Ludwig and were brought to the United States by Franklin P. Mall, who had studied with Ludwig in 1885–86 (Fleming 1954; Jarcho 1959). When Mall returned to the United States he became a professor of anatomy at the University of Chicago, and he began to advocate for a full-time system for the clinical faculty. He subsequently went to Johns Hopkins and continued his agitation there (Flexner and Flexner 1966:300–01). In 1902, Llewellys F. Barker, a colleague of Mall's at Hopkins, left to take the chair in anatomy at Chicago, and on February 28, 1902 in a speech before the Western alumni of Hopkins, he made the notion of a full-time plan the basis of his talk (Barker 1942). The speech was widely reviewed in the medical journals and stimulated some interest in this plan in the foundations. Gates heard about the speech and, through President Harper of Chicago, received an interview with Barker. In his autobiography Gates recalled: "From the time of my interview with Dr. Barker I became a hearty advocate of this idea" (1977:231).

It is not difficult to understand Gates's enthusiasm for a full-time plan. As previously noted, Gates believed that medical research would be able to find the cure for all diseases, or be able to prevent them. At the same time he believed that most practicing physicians were charlatans who preyed upon a naive and unsuspecting public. Gates saw the mission of the Rockefeller

A System of Scientific Medicine

philanthropies in medicine as turning it into a science and making its practitioners scientists. Scientists, he felt, should devote their entire attention to research and training future scientists. Any diversions or deviations from full-time research were violations of the code of honor of scientists and would have an inhibiting effect on making discoveries and finding cures. To the extent that physicians engaged in the private practice of medicine, medical progress through research slowed up.

Gates's first step in this regard came with the planning of a hospital for the Rockefeller Institute. Gates had written into the charter, with the approval of Simon Flexner and William Welch, both of whom were laboratory scientists, that:

> "No person on the salaried staff of the Institute should receive pay for any outside practice, that the Institute should itself send no bills for service to any patients within or without its walls, or accept any remuneration; that when expert members of the staff were called into unavoidable outside consultation, as in the case of eminent public men, the Institute should not only make no charge and accept no fees but should itself pay all expenses. The penalty for violation of these provisions by the Institute was the forfeiture of the endowment given by Mr. Rockefeller." [Gates 1977: 231]

The hospital planned in 1906 opened in 1910 and thus became the first institution in America to work under the full-time clinical plan and have the stipulations for such a plan expressly written into its charter. Given the close connection between the Rockefeller Institute and Johns Hopkins Medical School at this time (Corner 1959; Shryock 1953), and Hopkins's position in the forefront of scientific medicine in America (a position further enhanced by the Flexner Report), it seems appropriate that the GEB would start its attempt to achieve a full-time system of clinical medicine at Hopkins. In fact, Gates said:

> "We aimed at nothing less than a wide reform in the teaching and ultimately in the practice of medicine and Hopkins was only the place of beginning. With the highest ideals, the highest requirements and the highest standard of any medical college in the country it offered the best starting point for medical reform." [Gates 1977: 232]

In 1909 Dr. Clemens von Pirquet of the University of Breslau,

The Full-time Plan

Germany, spent a year as a visiting professor of pediatrics at Johns Hopkins Medical School and Johns Hopkins Hospital. The officials of Hopkins decided that von Pirquet would make an ideal chairman of the pediatrics department, and Dr. von Pirquet let it be known that under the right circumstances, he would be willing to stay at Johns Hopkins. In November 1910, Dr. Welch wrote to Simon Flexner at the Rockefeller Institute in New York with the following message:

> "Mr. Blanchard Randall has received a letter from von Pirquet saying that you and your brother [Abraham] are informed about his wishes and conditions for returning to us. We are of course most desirous of securing him, and shall do all in our power. I believe that if we could secure an endowment, say of $200,000, for the chair and department of pediatrics, we could at last establish a clinical department on an ideal basis, that is on the basis of a laboratory department. Von Pirquet would fall into such an arrangement perfectly. The idea is to have at the head of such a clinical department a productive investigator, who would make his hospital work, his teaching and the conduct of research the main things. He could build up a great school of pediatrics and would be a great stimulus and inspiration to the country. The new children's hospital is approaching completion, and is admirable. Do you suppose that we could present this matter to Mr. Rockefeller, through Mr. Gates, Mr. Murphy and his advisors, with a prospect of interesting them?" [Chesney 1963:123]

There are several interesting aspects to this letter. First is the use of Simon Flexner as the New York-based contact person with the Rockefellers and their associates. Second is the fact that though Abraham Flexner was just a staff person on the Carnegie Foundation payroll, and engaged in a study of medical education in Europe, he was already involved in attempts to reshape medical education in the United States well in advance of his formal position.

In December, 1910 Welch paid a visit to Gates at his home in New Jersey. Ostensibly the subject under discussion was Rockefeller money to implement the full-time plan at Johns Hopkins. While no record of that meeting exists, shortly after the meeting Gates responded to Welch:

"Dear Dr. Welch: I have not forgotten the main subject of conversation on the occasion of your recent visit to my home, so delightful to me and to us all. Nor has my interest in medical education in the United States decreased, nor my belief that the Johns Hopkins Medical School should occupy in the future a position even more important than in the past. I am looking, therefore, with deep interest, I might almost say solicitude, for the estimate you are preparing of the needs of the institution. I should like to have this estimate cover two things: First, the necessary expense of furnishing an entrance class of 100 each year as good facilities throughout their course as the institution can now offer to an entering class of 50 each year. Second, the expense of conducting the institution in such a way that none of its professors (I speak now of the ultimate ideal) shall be permitted to make anything beyond the merest nominal charge for consultation or other service. I am looking to secure, you perceive, the best possible teaching in the various departments — teaching uncomplicated with professional work outside, the model being the very best of the European schools and the best European practice and spirit." [Chesney 1963:131–32]

Welch responded to this letter a few days later and noted the enormity of the task that was now before him. He told Gates that it would take from ten days to two weeks to prepare the necessary information, although it could be done more quickly if there were any serious need. He also noted that the amount of money required to accomplish what Gates suggested would be very large. Gates replied to Welch in the following manner:

"I have your kind letter of January 8th; also your letter announcing that you will be with us on January 25th. We shall then have an opportunity, I hope, to go over the questions that we are studying, in more detail. It seems to me that the thing for us to do is to figure out now the ideal thing, whatever it may come to and however appalling the financial total. This will include the enlargement of the Hospital as well as the enlargement of other facilities. If we cannot compass so large an undertaking all at once, or if we cannot compass it at all, we can still have it before us and can build toward it so that everything that we shall do will mean progress toward a definite chosen end, and nothing that we shall do will be inconsistent with it. Let us, therefore, picture to ourselves the ideal and however little we do, work at least in that direction and consistently with it. I will agree not to be discouraged at your figures. Your letter prepares me in advance." [Chesney 1963:133–34]

During his visit to Gates on January 25, 1911, Welch gave Gates the estimates that had been requested. Gates wrote Welch on January 30 to say: "I have been reading over and thinking over these estimates that you left with me. The job they offer is, I am afraid, too big a one for me to tackle at this period in my life." (Chesney 1963:34). It was at this point apparently that Abraham Flexner was interviewed by Gates and sent down to Baltimore to prepare a formal report for the GEB.

By his own account, Flexner spent three weeks in Baltimore. His 25-page report to Gates recommended that $1,500,000 be given to Johns Hopkins Medical School to allow it to reorganize the departments of medicine, surgery, obstetrics, and pediatrics on a full-time basis. Additionally, Flexner recommended that the size of the school be reduced to 250 students and that $40,000 be allocated to the rebuilding of the Hunterian laboratory, which primarily housed animals and served as a surgical laboratory. Flexner, in his autobiography, said that Gates was favorably impressed by the report and prepared to act on it but that Flexner himself urged Gates to submit the report to Dr. Welch and to the Trustees of Johns Hopkins, "in order that the application might come from the university if the medical faculty and university trustees wished to act" (Flexner 1960:113). At the end of March 1911, Flexner returned to Baltimore to present his report to Welch and the trustees of Johns Hopkins and returned to New York the next day. Flexner noted that on April 2, 1911 he wrote the following note to his wife:

> "Mr. Gates has just called me up. 'I have just finished reading your report,' he said. 'I can hardly find words to express my satisfaction and delight. I am more than satisfied. It is a model. I have occasion to read many reports, but when I have read anything like that I can hardly recall, etc., etc., etc.' He talked a stream; I cannot recall it; my head fairly reeled, for he's going to do it my way! He asked, 'Will they have the backbone to cut the school, to reorganize it, etc.?' I said I thought so, if we furnished a little stiffening. 'All right,' he said, 'we look to you to steer it. Now I want Mr. Murphy and John D.

Jr. to read the report and then they and you and I will have a conference. That's the way to study an educational institution.' More etc.'s, etc.'s, etc.'s. We talked for ten minutes, he doing most of it, and thus it ran." [Flexner 1960:114]

This letter is most interesting because it is so anomalous to the public image of Flexner, the one that he created. That he put it in his autobiography therefore is puzzling indeed. Several issues stand out from this letter:

1 If Gates and the staff had already read the report when Flexner first came back from Baltimore, why would Gates call him after he was expressly sent down to discuss the report with the trustees to tell him he liked it?
2 It is strange that Flexner referred to the recommendation of the report as doing it "my way" when in fact that very recommendation had been discussed by Welch and Gates previously.
3 Gates made no mention of this phone call in his memoirs.
4 The basis for this second trip to Hopkins was so that it would not seem as if the GEB was forcing this money on the Medical School. It is not clear from the historical record if Welch acted as if he knew nothing about the report but agreed with it or if he informed the trustees that it was his idea in the first place.

After the meeting with the Trustees and Welch, the news of the recommendations within the report became known around the Medical School. Opposition to the report was fast and furious and ultimately delayed implementation of the full-time plan for over two years. The next section shall explore more fully the recommendations of the report, the new Flexner Report and its impact on the Hopkins faculty and on American medicine in general.

The struggle for the full-time plan at Johns Hopkins Medical School

As noted above, the full-time plan was supported by laboratory scientists who resented the high consulting incomes of clinical physicians. Whatever social value the full-time plan might hold, it is imperative to appreciate this ideological basis to its emergence.

The Full-time Plan

It is thus not insignificant that the full-time plan emerged first at the home of the laboratory scientists, the Rockefeller Institute, an institution dominated by laboratory scientists with only a handful of clinicians. Due to the extremely close ties between the Rockefeller Institute and the Johns Hopkins Medical School, there was a certain natural flow from one institution to the other, and it is not surprising that Hopkins was to be the first large-scale institution to attempt a full-time plan. The advisors to Gates and the other members of the Rockefeller organization were laboratory scientists who had trained at Hopkins and had graduated or migrated to full-time staff positions at the Rockefeller Institute or were on the Board of Directors of the Rockefeller Institute.

Because the laboratory scientists were in favor of the full-time plan does not mean that the clinicians saw merit in it. Indeed, they were strongly and vociferously opposed to it. To the clinician, the full-time plan would mean markedly reduced income, reduced public reputation, and in general reduced chances for more worldly success. It was because of the opposition of the clinicians that it became necessary to have the Board of Trustees of Johns Hopkins approve the Rockefeller grant. It was feared that the more famous clinicians might leave Hopkins, but that it might also seem as if the foundation was forcing this unwanted system on a medical school which desperately needed money.

As a result of his Carnegie Foundation report in 1910, Abraham Flexner gained much public attention and renown as the leading expert on medical education reform in the United States. He had acknowledged Hopkins as the leading medical school in the United States. Although he had not mentioned the full-time plan in his report, he was the obvious choice to help implement this new approach to medical educational organization in the United States. Again, it must be mentioned that his brother, Simon Flexner, was the protegé of Dr. Welch and was the Director of the Rockefeller Institute. Abraham was thus in an ideal position to attempt to implement this new system that was so dear to the heart of Gates, who saw it as a mechanism to increase the efficiency of medical research.

From the discussions between Welch and Gates prior to Abraham Flexner's trip to Johns Hopkins and from Gates's own

A System of Scientific Medicine

autobiographical writings, the purpose of Flexner's trip was to prepare a report that would advocate for a full-time clinical system. It seems that the strategy was to have Welch and Simon Flexner garner support among the laboratory scientists; have the GEB money available at any time as a financial inducement; have a willing candidate for at least one of the full-time positions on hand (Dr. von Pirquet); and have a report done that would appear objective but would forcefully advocate for the full-time plan. Perhaps what was not foreseen in this larger strategy was the vehemence and antagonism of the clinical faculty to this arrangement, although it is possible that it was Flexner's report that led to the battles that were to ensue and which will be described below.

Flexner's report was ostensibly a review of the financial position of the Johns Hopkins Hospital and Medical School and a consideration of three possible options for spending the proposed $1 million that the GEB was prepared to give the school. The options were:

— Option 1: Reduce the size of the school to 250; rebuild the Hunterian laboratory and endow it; place the departments of medicine, surgery, pediatrics, psychiatry, and women's clinic (gynecology and obstetrics) on a full-time basis.
— Option 2: Reduce the size of the school to 250; rebuild the Hunterian laboratory and the dispensary; build new buildings for pharmacology, a library and offices; create a department of bacteriology and hygiene.
— Option 3: Leave the school at 400 students; use the money in somewhat different amounts for the buildings described in option 2.

Were the report simply a discussion of internal finances and recommended options, the results might have been different. The tone for which Flexner won so much acclaim in his 1910 Report, was to create a much different situation in this 1911 Report.

The 1911 Report

Flexner began this report by describing the financial situation of the different departments within the medical school. His discus-

The Full-time Plan

sion of the laboratory departments is notable for the high praise that they received. He cited the great researchers that worked there at the time and had worked there previously; the important discoveries that had been made and were being made; the devotion of the faculty to teaching and research. In all, according to Flexner, they suffered only from a shortage of space or from too many students.

The hospital was reviewed next, and in this section Flexner noted that the pay wards of the hospitals did not contribute to the cross-subsidization of charity care as they had been designed, but rather were a drain on the hospital when viewed through a stepped-down cost accounting methodology. Flexner said:

> "The pay wards are thus an obvious convenience and advantage to the small number of professors privileged to use them, and they are practically full all of the time, with a waiting list, except in the summer. The tendency to fill them with patients who come to these physicians personally and not to the hospital as such has been developed by those to whom it has been a source of large income. The class of patients who used to pay the hospital a moderate fee in addition to room and board has been largely eliminated. The hospital has tied up more than $200,000 in buildings which it maintains chiefly as an accommodation to certain physicians and surgeons who, without risk or responsibility, can send thither private patients, for whom they procure, without expense to themselves, excellent care and from whom they collect large fees. I say 'chiefly', not wholly; for in some instances the patients in the pay wards are scientifically interesting and not financially profitable: occasionally their expenses are paid by the clinicians interested in them. For patients of this latter class, it is necessary that suitable accommodations be provided—but not necessarily separate buildings." [Chesney 1963:297]

Flexner described the finances of the hospital staff and then discussed the clinical departments. It was in this section of his report that the truly inflammatory remarks occurred as can be seen from the following excerpts:

> "As contrasted with the instructors on the laboratory side, the clinical staff has been on the whole less productive and less devoted. The instructors do not devote their time to science and education,— indeed, only a few of them devote any considerable part. ... Not

only has productive work been sacrificed to private professional engagements,—routine teaching and hospital work go by the board when a large fee is in prospect. Classes are turned over to subordinates in order that the chief may leave town to see patients, not because they are scientifically interesting, but because they are pecuniarily worth while. The meagreness of original output and the conditions existing in the private wards, as set forth above, are not independent of each other: they are both traceable to one cause, namely, the displacement of science and education by business." [Chesney 1963: 299]

Whether it was necessary to state the case for full-time through the disparagement of the clinical faculty is of no real importance. The clinical faculty would have been against the plan no matter how elegantly they had been flattered by this review. In Bulletin Number Four, Flexner had been able to overstate his case and he exaggerated somewhat without fear of repercussion because he was on the side of "progressive" institutions and had the support of the AMA. Flexner's second report for Gates about Johns Hopkins, which was expected to be a tactful, dispassionate and carefully worded appraisal of pros and cons, was the exact opposite. It was a hatchet job, pure and simple.

News of Flexner's report quickly spread around the medical school and the decision to have the proposal for a full-time system ratified by the Johns Hopkins Board of Trustees made the substance of the report, as well as the form, subject to public discussion. The most serious criticism was that rendered by Sir William Osler, the most distinguished of the Hopkins faculty, who had left to become Regius Professor of Medicine at Oxford University in England. Osler was so well respected, and his opinions carried so much weight, that his objections to Flexner's study became the focus of all discussion. It should be remembered that much as the Rockefeller people were in the thrall of laboratory scientists like Welch and Simon Flexner, it was Osler who had inspired Gates to think about scientific medicine in the first place. Osler addressed his letter to President Remsen of Johns Hopkins but also sent copies to people at the Hospital and the Medical School. He started out with the following:

"As an Angel of Bethesda he [Flexner] has done much good in troubling our fish-pond, as well as the general pool. The Report as a whole shows the advantage of approaching a problem with an unbiased mind, but there are many mistakes from which a man who knows the profession from the outside only could not possibly escape. It is a pity the Report was allowed to go out in its present form, as his remarks show a very feeble grasp of the clinical situation at the Johns Hopkins Hospital; but this is not surprising, and perhaps is not his fault, since he has not had the necessary training, nor, from the outside, could he get the knowledge to understand it. To say, for example, p. 14, as contrasted with the instructors in the laboratory side the clinical staff has been on the whole less productive and less devoted is simply not true. I deny the statement in toto—they have been more productive and quite as devoted. It is singularly unfortunate that he should not have been able to appreciate the work of the very men who have done as much, or more, than any others to build up the reputation of the school and to advance the best interests of the profession. To mention, out of many, only five names—the most stable on the staff!—Finney, Thayer, Bloodgood, Cushing and Cullen. It is not too much to say that these men have done scientific work of a standard equal to that of the highest of any laboratory men connected with the University; and in addition work which in practical import, in the translation of Science into the Art, no pure laboratory men could have done. To speak as Mr. Flexner does (p. 15 of the Report) of these men as blocking the line and preventing the complete development of a race or school is perhaps pardonable ignorance, but again it is certainly not true. Take away the share of the reputation of the Johns Hopkins Medical School—particularly in Europe, which knows chiefly the Hospital Bulletin and the Reports—contributed from the clinical side, and by the junior staff, and you leave it, in comparison, poor indeed! . . . It is hard to say which is the more prevalent on pp. 14 and 15 of the Report—unfairness or ignorance; but in either case gross injustice is done to the men who have made the Johns Hopkins Clinical School." [Chesney 1963:177-78]

Osler next addressed the question of research in clinical medicine and argued that such research can be done anywhere. He felt it was neither necessary nor desirable to do such research in a university hospital, the Hospital of the Rockefeller Institute, a purely clinical research institution being a case of an institution established strictly for purposes of research with no other competing aims. Moreover, turning the university hospital into a research institution would subvert the goals of training practitioners of medicine and confining the professors within the hospital would keep them out of touch with the profession:

> "The danger would be the evolution throughout the country of a set of clinical prigs, the boundary of whose horizon would be the laboratory, and whose only human interest was research, forgetful of the wider claims of a clinical professor as a trainer of the young, a leader in the multiform activities of the profession, and an interpreter of science to his generation, and a counsellor in public and private of the people, in whose interests after all the school exists. And, remember, what we do to-day the other schools will try to do to-morrow. ... The Trustees of the Hospital will do well to hesitate before handing over their magnificent 'plant' to a group of men to 'run' on the narrow lines of a research institute, and risk the termination of that close affiliation with the profession and the public which has made their clinical school the most potent distributor of scientific medicine in the United States." [Chesney 1963:180]

All this was Osler's preface. He then addresses the real object of his anger relative to the Report, the implication that the clinicians were profiting financially from the current system. He said: "Do not be led away by the opinions of the pure laboratory men, who have no knowledge of the clinical situation and its needs" (p.181):

> "Against the sin of prosperity, which looms large in Mr. Flexner's Report (p.17), the clinical professor must battle hard. I was myself believed to be addicted to it; but you will be interested to know, and I would like the Trustees of the Hospital to know, that I took out of Baltimore not one cent of all the fees—none of which came from hospital patients—I received in the sixteen years of my work. The truth is, there is much misunderstanding in the minds, and not a little nonsense on the tongues, of the people about the large fortunes made by members of the clinical staff. At any rate, let the University and Hospital always remember with gratitude the work of one 'prosperous' surgeon, whose department is so irritatingly misunderstood by Mr. Flexner. I do not believe the history of medicine presents a parallel to the munificence of our colleague Kelly to his clinic. ... There are other points which I should like to discuss, but this letter

is already too long. To one I must refer. If there is to be a New Model and a Self-denying Ordinance, under which the clinical professors are to live laborious days and scorn the delights of the larger life, let them come in on a University basis. If a man's value in the open market is to be considered, do not insult him by offering $7,500, as suggested in Alternative Scheme I, but, as laboratory men, let them be content with salaries which are thought good enough for men just as good. ... Take the money by all means, but use it: (1) to reduce the number of students, (2) to re-arrange the laboratories in accordance with Alternative Scheme II. But, lastly and chiefly, divert the ardent souls who wish to be whole-time clinical professors from the medical school in which they are not at home to the Research Institutes to which they properly belong, and in which they can do their best work." [Chesney 1963:181-83]

Osler's penultimate paragraph appears to have come more from his heart than the other parts of his letter. He wrote:

"We are all for sale, dear Remsen. You and I have been in the market for years, and have loved to buy and sell our wares in brains and books—it has been our life. So with institutions. It is always pleasant to be bought, when the purchase price does not involve the sacrifice of an essential ... but in Alternative Scheme I we chance the sacrifice of something that is really vital, the existence of a great clinical school organically united with the profession and with the public. These are some of the reasons why I am opposed to the plan as likely to spell ruin to the type of school I have always felt the Hospital should be and which we tried to make it—a place of refuge for the sick poor of the city—a place where the best that is known is taught to a group of the best students—a place where new thought is materialized in research—a school where men are encouraged to base the art upon the science of medicine—a fountain to which teachers in every subject would come for inspiration—a place with hearty welcome to every practitioner who seeks help—a consulting centre for the whole country in cases of obscurity. And it may be said, all these are possible with whole-time clinical professors. I doubt it. The ideals would change, and I fear lest the broad open spirit which has characterized the school should narrow, as teacher and student chased each other down the fascinating road of research, forgetful of those wider interests to which a great hospital must minister." [Chesney 1963:182]

While the above represented Osler's formal correspondence

about the Flexner Report, he also engaged in a good deal of informal correspondence addressing the same matters. Thus in a letter to Welch on May 23, 1911 Osler said:

> "What a time you must be having over this question of whole time clinical men! Cushing tells me I am quoted on both sides. It is difficult to give an opinion, not having heard the proposal. If, as Kelly mentioned in a letter, the salaries would be fixed at 7500 dollars, it would spell ruin to the Hospital. You could, perhaps get the good men for a few years for that, but they would flit off, inevitably. On the other hand if the Trustees paid liberal salaries of 15 to 20 thousand dollars they could always command the best men, and I would be strongly in favour of it. ... I think Hurd and some of the Trustees have a very exaggerated idea of the large incomes made by the clinical professors. I think I mentioned to Barker in a letter I did not find it hard to spend every cent of the income I made from patients in the 16 years I was at the Hospital, and of course a good deal of that went in a sort of legitimate advertising of the Hospital, just such as you have done so much in the exercise of hospitality, and to use the expressive phrase of the Arab—'kept a fat hand.' The question too is whether you could keep the public and the profession away from any man who had a reputation such as that of Kelly. It is different in England." [Chesney 1963:138–39]

This less hostile tone of course occurred before Osler had read the Flexner document. Therefore it suggests that had that report been written more tactfully, the breach between the clinical and laboratory faculty might not have been opened so widely and that Osler may have been more supportive of the concept of the full-time plan.

Full-time after Osler's letter

The vehemence of Osler's reaction to the full-time plan contributed to the deepening division within the Medical School faculty. As Dean of the School, Welch was fearful that if he rushed the plan through, a substantial portion of his faculty would leave. His approach was thus to proceed slowly and present the issue to people at Hopkins who might be persuaded to favor it, while letting the opposition weaken through faculty attrition. All this

The Full-time Plan

had to be explained to Gates and the others at the Rockefeller philanthropies for the delay was to be longer than two years. In a letter to Gates dated June 2, 1911 Welch attempted to explain the delay:

> "While the proposition to place the heads of certain clinical departments on the salaried, full time basis seems relatively simple, it would mark a most revolutionary change in existing conditions of medical education, if adopted. I know that you must have become impatient over the delay in hearing from me, but I have encountered great difficulties in obtaining from our Trustees such an expression of their views as would enable me to report definitely what they are willing to do in this matter. There has been considerable opposition to the plan both in the Faculty and among the Trustees, but as the plan is better understood and the arguments for it driven home, I believe that the opposition is lessening. Any attempt to force such revolutionary changes without full deliberation and weighing of the pros and cons would have been disrupting. I am sorry to say that Dr. Osler is strongly opposed to the plan, going so far in a letter received today as to say that it will wreck the hospital if we attempt it, at least on the basis of $7500 salaries for the chief physicians and surgeons. I am myself equally strong on the other side of the question, and I expect to be able to report to you favorably." [Chesney 1963:141]

On June 11, 1911 Welch sent to Gates a report on the proposal which in essence was the official position of the Johns Hopkins Medical School on the Flexner document. In this report, Welch outlined the main objections to Flexner's proposal:

> "The main objections urged against this proposal are: (1) the alleged difficulty or impossibility of securing and holding the best men for the positions with such salaries as could be contemplated, (2) the difficulty of keeping the public and the profession away from men with the reputations which these clinicians should have, and the loss to the community and medical practitioners by withdrawal of such men from outside practice, (3) the contention that limitation to practice within the hospital would deprive the teachers of opportunities and experience valuable to them in their own development, in their training of students destined to become practitioners and in promoting the interests of the medical school, and (4) the feeling, entertained even by some in sympathy with the general purposes of the plan, that the imposition of fixed rules and regulations upon the con-

duct and the use of the time of such men as would be entrusted with these clinical chairs would be harassing, improper and unnecessary." [Chesney 1963:145]

Welch answered these objections in the next section of his report to Gates. Briefly, he suggested that they could raise the salaries to $10,000 and keep the sums secret so that if it were necessary to pay someone more, it could be done. Welch felt that once the full-time plan were in place for several years, physicians would come to think of it as the norm, rather than the exception. He also thought that by relieving the new chiefs of service of administrative responsibilities, they would have more time to practice real medicine and feel less like employees. Welch had already noted that the Flexner proposals are "novel and even revolutionary in character" and that the full-time proposal

"involves such radical changes in conditions which now exist and have always existed in medical schools both here and in Europe that entire agreement of opinion as to the wisdom of the change is not to be expected. Nor can the plan be carried out without some hardship to individuals and some disturbance of personal relations. These are among the reasons why it has been deemed necessary or expedient to allow full time for deliberation and discussion and to endeavor to bring about a situation where the changes can be effected with the least possible disturbance of the exceptionally harmonious relations which have always existed in our faculty." [Flexner and Flexner 1966:309-10]

Famous clinicians around the turn of the century were wealthy. It is estimated that Osler made $40,000 in the year 1902 (Harrell 1973:545-68). The surgeons Halstead and Kelly also received large sums. While famous clinicians were not that numerous, the most distinguished grouping was found at Hopkins in this time period and they had to be among the wealthiest. Clearly, they would be skeptical of a system which would substantially reduce their incomes.

Flexner's report to Gates estimated salaries for the chiefs of services to be $7,500. When the plan was finally approved this amount was raised to $10,000, but it was still substantially below the amounts the most distinguished clinicians were accustomed to receiving. In his letter, Osler protested the implication that he

The Full-time Plan

had become wealthy at the expense of his research and teaching duties, as Flexner had suggested in the report. Osler maintained that the clinical physicians were not wealthy; that many re-invested much of their income in the hospital or medical school and helped to improve the facilities; and that he in particular had not gotten rich from his private clients. Welch's response to Gates suggested that younger clinicians would eventually become accustomed to making less money and hence would grow to accept the salary as normal.

The clinicians feared that locked within the hospital they would lose contact and experience with diseases that were not found inside the hospital. They feared that they would fall into the diagnostic fallacy that medical sociologists now refer to as "selective bias" (Freidson 1970: 270–71). Other reservations included the concern that clinicians in the community would not be able to avail themselves of the greater diagnostic capability of the full-time physicians and that the ultimate sufferers would be the patients who did not want to receive their care in the hospitals. Moreover, the clinicians recognized that restriction to the hospital would limit their abilities to train students for anything other than hospital diagnosis and hence would make them less effective teachers to those students who were not destined to become hospital clinicians.

The clinicians resented the proletarianization that was being foisted upon them. In many cases, they were independently wealthy and were not dependent upon the "bureaucrats" in either the hospitals or the foundations for their livelihoods. The laboratory scientists needed the foundations, for it was through the foundations' largesse and support that they maintained their positions. If they did not follow the mandates of the foundations, they might well be without jobs. On the other hand, the clinicians were not dependent upon the hospitals or the foundations. They could establish their own hospitals or maintain private practices and they had the support of the community.

The establishment of the full-time plan in medical schools probably represented the first time that the philanthropic foundations had dealt with a social grouping that was not dependent upon them for their livelihoods. The clinicians were in a different position *vis-à-vis* impoverished university professors or southern farmers since they had more options and their independence was much easier to maintain.

The advocates of the full-time plan predicted tremendous advances in clinical research resulting from the devotion of the best clinicians completely to research and teaching. They saw outside practice, even the teaching of future practitioners, to be a distraction from the important needs of medicine (i.e. research) and the promotion of a discredited commercialism in medicine from practitioners who were not scientists. They were clearly promoting a hospital-based medicine. Gates along with Rockefeller, Jr., who shared his perspective, clearly saw the matter in this light. In a memorandum to Rockefeller, Sr. advocating his giving $1,200,000 to Hopkins, and hand delivered with a personal introduction by Rockefeller, Jr., Gates said the following when discussing the last two (clinical) years of the Hopkins medical school:

> "These two years introduce the student for the first time to the bedside of the sick. They are the clinical years. The professors in these departments, while chosen originally for their scientific attainments, very quickly found themselves solicited to extensive practice, partly because of their skill, partly because of the fame of the institution with which they are associated as Professors. Wealthy patients from distant parts of the country, ready to pay any price for their services, embarrassed them with demands upon their time. As a consequence, in the course of a few years the professors in the clinical department of the college have become widely celebrated practitioners of medicine and surgery and overwhelmed with demands from outside patients. They have filled the wards of the hospital with these patients. They have in addition in some instances built private hospitals of their own. They have been able to charge and collect enormous fees for their services and their incomes have grown to enormous proportions, the least of them probably receiving an income scarcely less than that of the President of the United States, and from that up to amazing figures. The consequences of this have been practically the same as with the other schools of medicine. These professors have little time to give to their classes. Calls have taken them away from the recitations room for days or weeks at a time. They have had little time for research. They have made few contributions to the science of

medicine as compared to their confrères of the first two years [the laboratory years] and they have set before the classes of Johns Hopkins the evil example of commercialism in the medical profession and their lives have stimulated the avarice of the students, while not contributing as they should contribute to their scientific and philanthropic enthusiasm." [Flexner and Flexner 1966: 311–12]

It is interesting to note, in the light of this letter, that these thoughts did not prohibit Gates from summoning Dr. Barker from Hopkins to attend to him at his home in New Jersey during an illness (Gates to Rockefeller, Jr., June 4, 1909, Rockefeller Family Archives). Towards the end of this memorandum, Gates continued:

"It is, of course, a revolutionary suggestion promising to place medical education on a height of disinterested service never yet reached. It cannot be effected without serious disturbances of vested interests. Several of the professors with large incomes will either have to resign from the institution to private practice, or else their incomes will be reduced to half and in some instances perhaps one-tenth of what they have been. These men do not accept this situation without pretty serious heart searchings. Some of them are prepared to make the sacrifice, perceiving it to be in the interests of science and humanity. Others will take their places, not with the sheep, but with the goats on the left hand and continue medicine as a commercial pursuit, disassociated from the college."

By starting at the most influential school, the GEB also began the full-time plan at the school with the wealthiest clinicians, the ones least likely to endorse the new plan. If the GEB had started with a lesser school, they might have had an easier time, but clearly they were interested in establishing the model at the top and letting it filter down. They seem to have underestimated the resentment and resistance of the clinicians.

The imbroglio over the full-time plan was resolved in 1913 when Welch, as acting President of the Johns Hopkins University, wrote to the GEB requesting funds for setting up the departments of medicine, surgery, and pediatrics on a full-time basis (Flexner and Flexner 1966: 324) The fighting had died down after the original fracas in 1911, however while the infighting may have ended, the problems still remained. The position of professor of medicine was first offered by Welch to Lewellys Barker, one of the original advocates of the plan.

He turned down the offer because he could not afford to give up his lucrative private practice with the expenses of children in college and a sick family (Barker 1942). The next offer was made to William S. Thayer, who also refused the position. Finally it was offered to Theodore Janeway, a professor of medicine at Columbia University. Within three years, though, Janeway gave up the position in part because of financial need and in part because of disillusionment with the full-time system (Flexner and Flexner 1966: 325–326).

A second problem had to do with the contract authorizing the full-time system between the GEB and Johns Hopkins University. Care had to be taken to ensure that it was Johns Hopkins who requested the money for the purposes outlined and that the only action of the GEB was to agree financially to support the proposal. Since foundations were coming under increasing criticism from the public and the government for manipulative practices, the foundation wanted it made clear, on the record, that it was simply responding to a request from the University. Thus, in anticipation of a new attack on the philanthropic foundations, the following statement was made:

> "On the request of the faculties of Johns Hopkins, Washington and Yale universities, the Board had provided money to organize full-time staffs in the Departments of Medicine, Surgery and Pediatrics. The plans for this reorganization were drafted by the medical faculty of Johns Hopkins University, who have complete responsibility for the innovation; the General Education Board simply provided the necessary means." [General Education Board 1914: 166–68]

This policy was to be followed at all the other schools that changed to the full-time system.

Finally, while the press reaction was generally favorable, having been given the story either by Welch or the GEB, and not being fully aware of the issues at hand, the medical press was much less enthusiastic about the new system. While some at first reacted solely to the announcement in terms which indicated they were glad to get new money into medicine, most of the medical journals came out strongly against the system by 1914. The leader in this criticism was the *Journal of The American Medical Association* *(JAMA)* which published a long series of critiques on the "Hopkins Plan". The Council on Medical Education of the AMA established a committee of clinicians to study the full-time plan. This committee concluded that the plan was not the "ideal". The Council, feeling this was not sufficient criticism, carried on the fight against the plan, becoming more involved as the number of schools with the full-time plan increased (Flexner and Flexner 1966: 322 -24).

12
The Full-time Plan Expands to Other Schools

The second school to adopt the full-time plan was Washington University (Munger 1968). Robert Brookings, a millionaire who owned warehouses in St. Louis, was a trustee of Washington University and had taken a personal interest in its medical school. After Flexner's first visit to the school in 1909, his report notes described Washington University as "a little better than the worst ... but absolutely inadequate in every essential respect" (Munger 1968: 358). Brookings wrote to Henry Pritchett, President of the Carnegie Foundation, and demanded a full explanation. Flexner was sent back to St. Louis to defend his description of the school and succeeded in convincing Brookings that the school was as bad as his report had made it out to be. Brookings pledged to make the school the best in the Mid-west. When the Flexner Report was released in 1910, Washington University received a very favorable notice.

After hearing of the Hopkins full-time grant, Brookings applied within a month for a similar grant for Washington University. With the aid of the GEB, Washington University became the second school in the country to adopt the full-time system (Munger 1968: 367–69).

Over the next several years, grants were awarded to Yale, Rochester, Vanderbilt, University of Chicago, and Harvard. During the 1920s, money was appropriated to such schools as Cornell, Columbia, University of Iowa, and McGill for full-time systems (Flexner 1960:161–79). While each of the individual dramas surrounding the introduction of the full-time system is fascinating, certain stories highlight the dynamics of philanthropic foundations and the counter-revolt of the medical profession. Examples of a few of these cases follow.

While negotiations were still going on between the GEB and Johns Hopkins, the GEB invited Harvard University to submit an application for a full-time clinical system (Brown 1979:166). While Hopkins was the leading school of scientific medicine in the United States at the time, Harvard had the highest prestige and its clinical faculty represented the upper class of Boston social circles. Independently wealthy and catering to the needs of the Boston elite, the Harvard clinicians were not interested in giving up their consulting incomes and practices. Yet, it would be a tremendous coup for the advocates of the full-time plan to be able to claim Harvard as one of theirs. The former President of Harvard, Charles Eliot, long an ardent supporter of scientific medicine, and also an important Trustee of the GEB, represented the interests of the clinicians in the GEB boardroom. Eliot claimed, rightfully, that the GEB's insistence on the absolute exclusion of private income as a contractual stipulation violated the Board's established policy of non-interference with the internal operations of recipient agencies. Eliot argued that the full-time plan asked the Board to do just this and that therefore the Board should not insist upon strict adherence to the plan through legal contract. The full-time contracts that had been signed by Johns Hopkins and Washington University contained clauses that mandated that the GEB money be returned if strict full-time plans were not in operation. Gates had insisted on such contractual language from his earliest days with the Rockefeller organization, feeling that without it, the foundation would have no influence after making its grants. As time wore on, the Harvard clinicians remained adamant in their refusal to accept a strict notion of full-time and demanded a certain amount of private practice. The "Harvard Plan" essentially allowed full-time clinical professors to retain a small percentage of their time for an independent consulting practice. This became the precursor for the dominant full-time plan in the United States today, known as the geographic full-time system.

A similar situation occurred when the GEB attempted to install a full-time system at Columbia University. It brought the Carnegie Foundation into the fracas and Henry Pritchett became an adversary to the notion of strict adherence clauses in the GEB contracts (Brown 1979: 172–74). By 1925, the GEB formally removed the noncompliance clause from the full-time contract.

The American Medical Association and the full-time plan

As noted above, when the full-time plan was first introduced at Johns Hopkins in 1913, the general reaction of the medical community, as evidenced by the AMA, was one of mild support and wait-and-see attitude. By 1914, they were clearly against the plan. Arthur Bevan, as Chairman of the Council on Medical Education, led the attack on the full-time plan. He started his critical attacks in 1912, while the plan was still under discussion. In a letter to Abraham Flexner on January 9, 1912, he said:

> "The absurd plan which has been discussed at Johns Hopkins of putting men in charge of our clinical departments who are to be paid very large salaries and who are not to be permitted to receive any compensation in private practice, or if they do, to have this compensation paid to the treasury of the university cannot be too severely condemned, and must have arisen in the minds of men, probably laboratory men, who are not familiar with modern clinical medicine." [Flexner Papers, Library of Congress]

And to Henry Pritchett on January 10, 1912:

> "I remember your telling me the interesting story of the reasons which led up to the establishment of the Carnegie Foundation, the difficulty in keeping the best brains in engineering and other departments in our teaching faculties. I am afraid if the Johns Hopkins plan which I refer to in my letter to Mr. Flexner [above] is generally adopted that it will be impossible for the medical schools to keep the best brains in medicine in the teaching positions." [Flexner Papers, Library of Congress]

By 1914, Bevan denounced the plan as "grotesque" and the "plan of a layman" (A. Flexner to H. Judson, December 29, 1914, Rockefeller Foundation Archives). As more schools shifted over

Full-time Plan Expands to Other Schools

to the full-time plan, the criticism became more intense and personal. Bevan and other leaders of the AMA appealed to Pritchett to use his and the Carnegie Foundation's influence to stop the GEB from implementing its plan (Penfield 1967: 214–15). On November 11, 1919, Pritchett wrote to Wallace Buttrick, President of the GEB:

> "I never looked carefully at the contract between the General Education Board and the Johns Hopkins University and Chicago University until after I was talking with you and Flexner today. I must confess I was rather staggered by them. These contracts laid down a stated policy for conducting a medical school which the Board approves and then in a formal contract the universities bind themselves to carry out these policies, and agree not to change them except by permission of the General Education Board, and in case they change without such permission the universities agree to return the money. Such a contract binding a university to a fixed policy laid down by the giver of the money seems to me a dangerous thing. If these contracts were made public I am sure it would bring down on all educational foundations no less than on universities themselves severe criticism. It seems to me a dangerous policy for those who administer trust funds to adopt." [Carnegie Foundation Files]

Buttrick replied on November 21, 1919:

> "I fear that you failed to notice that the preamble to the contract with Johns Hopkins University distinctly recites that the policy was proposed to us by the Trustees and medical faculty of the university and that the terms of the contract were such as they themselves asked for. The General Education Board has no fixed policy regarding medical education, and certainly it did not presume to lay down a policy for the Medical School of the Johns Hopkins University. After this work was inaugurated three other universities sought our aid on similar terms and our pledges were made in accordance with their requests and suggestions. In fact, the contracts were drawn under the supervision of their own legal advisors." [Carnegie Foundation Files]

Pritchett responded to Buttrick as follows:

> "I do not think the preamble to which you refer greatly alters the situation. Even though the trustees of the university came to one of

the foundations and proposed a policy, it is in my judgement a very questionable proceeding to draw up a contract binding them to such a policy which they may not change without the consent of the corporation giving the funds. Particularly does this seem a dangerous proceeding when coupled with the condition that the failure to accept this outside control involves the return of the funds. Looking at the contract even in light of your statement it seems to me to be open to a very serious objection and I am inclined to think that it will sometime in the future bring upon all of us a kind of criticism difficult to answer." [November 25, 1919, Carnegie Foundation Files]

In the case of Columbia University, the contract was actually put to the test. The medical faculty of Columbia, which had fought the imposition of the contract but finally accepted it, later voted to modify the contract by allowing the full-time professors to accept outside fees (Brown 1979:173). The Columbia situation received wide attention from the public as it involved large sums of money from the Rockefeller Foundation, the Carnegie Corporation and several other individual donors, along with the GEB all involved in the creation of the Columbia–Presbyterian Medical Center. After much infighting among board members of the GEB, it was decided not to force the issue and to allow Columbia's faculty to have its way. The clauses on returning the money were soon eliminated from future contracts.

In his autobiography, Gates concluded his chapter on the full-time plan with the following comments:

"At the time of this writing [1926–28] ten of the principal medical colleges in the United States have adopted full-time in whole or in part and there seems little doubt that had not our boards recently and as I think unwisely cancelled the legal obligation of the full-time restriction, the academic basis would in no long time have prevailed among medical colleges in the United States. Unfortunately, as the matter now stands, success is and as I think can be partial only." [1977: 233]

Medical systems in Europe

Despite the fact that advances were clearly being made in American medical education and research, the European medical schools and research institutes were still far superior to those in the United States. Many of the European institutes had suffered physical deterioration and most of the laboratory projects and research programs had been abandoned during the war for more pressing problems (Fosdick 1952:107-09). The foundations considered it essential that before aid be given to countries without medical education systems, the great systems of Western Europe and England must be rebuilt.

The Rockefeller Foundation took the opportunity to introduce variations of the full-time plan into the British schools and to emphasize the research ideal in medical education. While exact amounts are unattainable, it is certain that Britain received over $6 million; France $1½ million; Belgium $4½; Canada $10 million. In addition, significant amounts were given to medical schools in Brazil, Lebanon, Australia, and other areas of the Pacific (Fosdick 1952:109-22). While the Foundation tried hard to influence these countries to accept the full-time plan, the British rebelled and instituted a modified plan leaving two days a week for physicians to pursue private practice. The French were more hostile to the attempted imposition of full-time and turned down a gift of $12 million so they would not have to accept the restrictions.

What was clearly recognized was that medicine was not the property of one nation and that the best results in medical research came from large numbers of people studying the same problems. Medical research being spread over the world would have the same impact as it was hoped it would have on the United States. To be sure, the Foundation's officers also saw this philanthropy as a means of entry into Europe for more classic capitalist ventures. Thus Gates was able to say:

> "My next suggestion of possible aid to the nations of Western Europe is the investment of capital among the peoples impoverished by the Great War. This should be done by purchases of their public securities, to be paid for by the transfer of gold, which will also help to make stable their currencies. To be sure, this is straight business and not philanthropy at all. But just now it is for Western Europe more philanthropic than philanthropy. It will release local capital for local uses. It will set labor to work, turn the wheels of industry, develop natural resources, multiply exports, promote commerce. This

transfer of American capital to Europe is doing and will do more to restore the peace and prosperity of Europe than the League of Nations could do, even were America in it. An investment pure and simple, the field is inviting as philanthropy is of the best. Why not kill two birds with one stone?" [Gates 1927:5]

The Rockefeller Foundation was clearly infused with a sense of mission. They were in the envious position of having assets of over $100 million and virtually no restrictions on how or where to spend it. This was a period of increasing internationalization of United States capital, a process that first became obvious during the Spanish–American War. The World War provided an opportunity for American capital to buy into Europe at phenomenally low rates because of the European need for money at the end of the war. The foundation viewed itself as supporting and complementing that investment in and of capital by supporting services that would help to produce a stable labor force for European capital. Gates said, though it is not clear that he considered it to be hyperbole: "I sometimes think that for the real issue of mankind this [the Rockefeller Foundation] is by far the most important legislative body in the world and we as individuals here are weighted with the heaviest responsibilities" ("Tentative Suggestions as to World Strategy in Medicine", p.2, Rockefeller Foundation Archives).

By 1928, the GEB invested $60 million in medical education, almost entirely in support of the full-time clinical plan. The Board even went so far as to pass a resolution in 1914 stating: "The Board does not consider it expedient at present to aid medical education except insofar as it concerns the installation of full-time clinical teaching" (Fosdick 1962:159). By 1960, when the GEB was dissolved, it had spent over $94 million on medical education (28.9 per cent) out of a total of $325 million spent for all purposes (Fosdick 1962:172).

It has been estimated that when the contributions of local sources, alumni and other philanthropic sources are summed up, the total amount of money going strictly into medical education reform amounted to over $600 million (Fosdick 1962:172). The vision of Gates in the 1890s—for a system of scientific medicine

—was moving toward becoming a reality in the United States by the 1930s and also in the rest of the world.

Flexner, Gates, and scientific medical education

When the GEB was given its first large endowment supplement of $10 million in 1905, Gates drew up a set of policy principles for how this money was to be used. Foremost among these principles was that the money would not be used to support state or public universities and colleges. In a statement read to the Board on January 23, 1906, Gates said:

> "Unlike the Russian universities, which have been closed by the state from time to time, our state universities have never come into serious conflict with the power which controls them, doubtless because the Legislatures have been disposed to give, in this land of free speech, large freedom of instruction. But we know not what social paroxysms await us, and the higher agencies of education ought to be fortresses—impregnable fortresses of truth. If too great dependence on the populace for annual support is a possible weakness of our state universities, that fact becomes a powerful reason for endowing the private institutions. If the test should ever come, the power which will act most effectively to preserve the state institutions will be private and denominational colleges and universities amply endowed and holding and teaching truth whatever may be the passions of the hour, and ultimately directing popular opinion into right channels. Better yet and more probable, the private foundations everywhere numerous and free, will so enlighten and direct popular opinion at all times that there can never ensue a conflict between the democracy and its state universities."

Gates had other reasons for not wanting to give Foundation grants to the state universities:

1. The GEB should not create the impression that they were "buying" the state schools by giving them grants.
2. Because this was a period of considerable anti-trust activity on the part of the government, there was a sense that if the government were going to confiscate private revenues then it would be directed toward the governmental support of the schools.

3. Because of discussion about a national income tax (first discussed in the early 1890s and eventually implemented in 1913) there was a similar sense that if the government were going to take money from private organizations, it was foolish to give additional money back to the government through grants.

This policy regarding state universities was not unique to the GEB. The Carnegie Foundation also initially barred state universities from participating in its pension plan.

The trustees of the GEB approved Gates's policy statement which also called for grants to be given only for endowment and to be made only to schools in centers of populations. Regardless of this policy, in terms of day-to-day activities, these principles were violated as regularly as they were honored. In fact, Wallace Buttrick, President of the GEB, said on many occasions that "our one policy is to have no policy" (Flexner 1960:136).

The initial Board was largely composed of businessmen who presumably felt the same way about state universities and government confiscation of private profits as Gates did. In a letter to George Peabody dated November 20, 1911, Gates noted:

"It seems strange that Mr. Peabody in looking over the list of members of the Board could have imagined that Mr. Rockefeller could have gathered these gentlemen to 'throw new light on the important problems of education in this country.' Let us look at the personnel of the Board for a moment: Two of them were educated as Baptist ministers and their early years were spent in the pulpit; one is a great, successful merchant, now retired; two are authors, editors and publishers, widely intelligent as such men must be; two are bankers and railroad promoters—one retired; one might be called purely and simply a capitalist; one is a lawyer; two are or have been successful manufacturers; one is a great manufacturer now engaged in philanthropy. These gentlemen form two thirds of the Board, and absolutely control its policies ... It is easy to see that the purpose of the founder in getting together this mixed body of men, giving overwhelming preponderance to business men, was to fix the policies of this Board along the lines of successful experience and to put so much of the heavy ballast in the ship as to prevent its being carried away with the fads or new lights of any kind on the subject of education. He knew that successful business men would steer the ship along traditional lines and would not be carried out of their course by any temporary breeze or even by hurricanes of sentiment."

After the Senate hearings on the role of foundations in the wake of the Ludlow Massacre, many foundation boards and their policies began to change. Newer board members reflected the new "corporate liberalism" and attempted to work with the government rather than assuming it an implacable foe. Rockefeller, Jr., for example, took a more moderate posture *vis-à-vis* working with government than did his mentor Gates. In fact as more members of the Board began to reflect the friends and associates of the younger Rockefeller rather than the founder, the nature of the Board changed substantially. In particular the newer members of the Board were seemingly less impressed with the ancient oratorical style that Gates represented than were the more established Board members. These issues came to a head over discussions of the Board's policy on medical education.

In 1913, Abraham Flexner formally joined the staff of the GEB as secretary for medical education. His job was to select schools to be given a full-time grant and to secure local matching money for these grants. Flexner was made a member of the Board of Trustees in 1914. This is notable because it allowed a member of the staff to influence other Trustees and to vote on projects that he initiated. This was to bring Flexner into heated conflict with Gates as time went by.

When Abraham Flexner came to the GEB, his job was to spread the message of full-time far and wide. He took his job seriously and literally. He looked around the country for areas where full-time scientific medical care would thrive. His search was for medical schools that were amenable to educational improvement and upgrading and this search took him to the Mid-west. In this area of the United States, virtually all the medical schools were state supported schools. There were no private medical schools that were of sufficient quality to upgrade, nor were there any private universities willing to make a major effort to establish a medical school. In Bulletin Number Four, Flexner had talked about the need to upgrade the state institutions of the Mid-west as these were the only institutions capable of providing scientific

A System of Scientific Medicine

medical education.

Had Flexner simply been a staff member, his recommendations could have been voted down with little fuss. But as a Board member, his views had equal weight with other members and he was in a position to defend his own proposals. It must be noted that Flexner sought to build a system of scientific medicine in the most rational way that he knew, independent of the auspices of the medical school. He was not influenced by the ownership of the school because he was not involved with the larger issues of confiscation or income taxation that concerned the older members of the Board, for whom the question of auspice was of overriding significance no matter what violence it did to the rationality of a plan for systematic medical education.

The first major fight between Gates and Flexner came over Flexner's proposal to give money to the University of Iowa Medical School in 1922. Flexner sought $2½ million from the Rockefeller philanthropies to support the construction of a modern hospital and clinical setting on the site of the medical school. His basic argument to the Board was that Iowa was a progressive state that would match the grant and help to uplift medical education in that area.

Gates's strong opposition to this proposal was based on several points:

1 There was a surplus of physicians in the United States and therefore no need for new doctors and moreover no need for medical schools which turned out practitioners (rather than researchers) as Iowa did.
2 The real needs in medical education were in the area of medical research not clinical practice, a world-wide need especially in light of the destruction of medical schools in Europe during World War I.
3 Medical schools could only flourish in major cities or large population centers.
4 Any money that was not invested in research should be invested in prevention.

In addition Gates felt strongly that there was no reason to give money to a state school. He did not see how the GEB could refuse other state institutions once it gave money to Iowa. He was upset about the size of the grant, which would be more than was given to his favorite institutions, Hopkins and Harvard. He was also concerned that the money would build a hospital rather than change Iowa to a full-time clinical plan. Gates did not think that Iowa was a particularly distinguished school and did not think that the grant money would improve its reputation in the field.

Perhaps most strongly, he felt that the proper course for Iowa was not to appeal to an outside philanthropy but rather to go to the legislature to request support. If the legislature refused to grant the necessary funds, the next recourse for the state medical school was to canvass the state and in that manner obtain the cooperation and support of the entire populace in the efforts to upgrade medical education. Iowa, he felt, was a very wealthy state that did not need outside financial assistance. Gates felt very strongly that the first duty of a community was to its own health and medical care and that this was not a role that should be usurped by philanthropy without doing great damage to the internal structure and cohesion of the community.

When the Iowa grant was put before a meeting of the Board, the fighting was fast and furious. Gates orated for over three hours while Flexner spoke for less than twenty minutes. In the end, the Board voted with Flexner. Gates could never reconcile himself to this fundamental breach in his control over the Board. As long as he remained on the Board he continued to vote against every appropriation made for a grant to a state medical school. In every case he was on the losing side of the vote and in some cases the sole opposing vote.

When Flexner attempted to reconcile with Gates, the latter rebuffed him with the following letter on December 2, 1922:

> "I have made much of the Iowa matter and fought it hard not only because of its intrinsic importance but also and mainly because it has been presented by you as a sample of your future policy for the central west Alleghenies to the Rockies. This means as you stated specifically: A. Building up by preference the State Medical Schools as in Iowa; B. Giving them if necessary say half of the required sum, as in Iowa; C. Doing this utterly regardless of their wealth of financial ability as in Iowa; D. Doing this in the face of the obvious the

A System of Scientific Medicine

conceded fact these schools are controlled by the taxpayers, as in Iowa; E. Doing it in face of the fact, as in Iowa, that the taxpayer is not intelligent on the needs and cost of first class medical education; F. Doing it with no guarantee whatsoever of any sort of vertical uplift; G. Doing it without the least attempt to give Iowa the one supreme and simple thing Iowa needs—viz. illumination of the voter. If the Iowa programme could be accepted 'in principle' all these results follow. And more, I figure there are some 32 states that can present 'in principle' a better case than Iowa's. Why confine this policy to the Central West? The south has a far better claim. It is amazing. How *could* you! You have never squarely met one of my arguments."

For the rest of his life Gates continued to argue against this policy of granting money to state schools and to write letters to Rockefeller, Jr. complaining about the mistake he made when he allowed a staff member to join the Board. Both Gates and Flexner had clear conceptions of how a system of scientific medicine would develop. For Gates, the medical education system could not be separated from the larger political economy of the nation. His was a viewpoint that had had its time and place and was quickly losing its prominence on the American scene. For Flexner, his vision of a medical education system around the country was independent of factors other than his ability to interest trustees or local donors to give money to support scientific medicine. His was a viewpoint that would continue to be in the mainstream.

Abraham Flexner left the GEB Board on June 30, 1928 and went on to other ventures including the creation of the Lincoln School, an experiment in progressive education modelled on his old preparatory school in Louisville and much later he became the first Director of the Institute for Advanced Study in Princeton, New Jersey. Gates resigned from the Board of the GEB on December 31, 1928. He died on February 6, 1929.

The history of American medical education is incomplete unless the stories of both of these men and the organizations that they represented are told. Their dreams were for a system of scientific medical education in the United States and they helped to create the system that exists today.

As this narrative history has been related chronologically, it can be seen that the GEB's strategy was to proceed in a linear fashion. Through a series of calculated steps, the Board, representing major philanthropic interests, played a pivotal role in the development and expansion of medical education. The growing involvement through large financial contributions for specific projects and within carefully worded contracts has had an immeasurable impact on the field of medicine today. This growing involvement can be viewed as a series of three major movements or steps:

Step 1 was the creation of the Rockefeller Institute, a local venture which gave the Rockefeller organization some necessary exposure to and experience in the field of scientific medicine.

Step 2 in the growing GEB's involvement in the medical field began with the significant financial contributions to medical education and the reshaping of the field by influencing the reform of clinical teaching to emphasize research more fully. Through a redirected system of teaching scientific medicine, not only were the research capabilities of American scientists expanded but the gospel of scientific medicine was spread throughout the country. Through a process resembling osmosis, the graduates of the Rockefeller Institute, Johns Hopkins and other supported schools (including Washington University, Harvard, Yale, Rochester, Chicago, and Vanderbilt) soon began to spread out to other schools across the country, infiltrating those institutions with strong commitments to science and research rather than an emphasis on clinical practice alone.

Step 3 involved the sustained support and thereby the expansion of medical education not only to a few major institutions but beyond the elite private schools initially supported by foundation money. This continued involvement and expanded influence has had major influence on the medical field and created the system of scientific medical education that exists in the United States today.

Notes on the Archival Sources

This book makes use of documents, letters, memoranda, and reports drawn from a number of archival sources. While dates and correspondents have been included in the references, the individual collections from which documents have been drawn have been omitted.

The following listing of archives and the collections utilized should assist scholars and others who desire to extend this research.

Carnegie Foundation Archives, Carnegie Foundation, New York. (Archive files)

Council on Medical Education, American Medical Association, Chicago. (Minutes).

Oral History Research Collection, Columbia University, New York. (Abraham Flexner Interview)

Manuscript Division, Library of Congress, Washington. (Abraham Flexner Papers; Henry Pritchett Papers; Andrew Carnegie Papers)

Welch Medical Library, The Johns Hopkins University, Baltimore. (William H. Welch Papers; William Osler Papers)

Rockefeller Family Archives, Rockefeller Archives Center, Pocantico Hills, New York. (Gates Philanthropy; Educational Interests; Friends and Associates)

Rockefeller Foundation Archives, Rockefeller Archives Center, Pocantico Hills, New York. (Gates Papers)

Notes on the Archival Sources

Joseph Regenstein Library, University of Chicago, Chicago. (Presidential Papers; Harper Papers; Goodspeed Papers; J.D. Rockefeller Papers; Gates Papers)

References

Abel-Smith, B. (1964) *The Hospitals.* Cambridge: Harvard University Press.
Ackerknecht, E.H. (1948) Anticontagionism Between 1821 and 1867. *Bulletin of the History of Medicine* 22: 562-93.
Adamic, L. (1931) *Dynamite: The Story of Class Violence in America.* New York: Vintage.
American Medical Association, Council on Medical Education (1907) *Minutes.* Chicago: AMA.
Banta, H.D. (1971) Abraham Flexner—A Reappraisal. *Social Science and Medicine* 5: 655-61.
Barker, L. (1942) *Time and the Physician.* New York: G. Putnam.
Beard, C. and Beard, M. (1937) *The Rise of American Civilization.* New York: Macmillan.
Berliner, H.S. (1975) A Larger Perspective on the Flexner Report. *International Journal of Health Services* 5: 573-92.
    (1977) New Light on the Flexner Report. *Bulletin of the History of Medicine* 51: 603-09.
    (1982) Medical Modes of Production. In A. Treacher, and P. Wright, (eds) *The Problem of Medical Knowledge.* Edinburgh: University Press.
Berliner, H.S. and Salmon, J.W. (1979) Scientific Medicine and Holistic Health: The Naked and the Dead. *Socialist Review* 9: 31-52.
Billroth, T. (1924) *The Medical Sciences in the German Universities.*

New York: Macmillan.
Bonner, T.N. (1957) *Medicine in Chicago: 1850–1950.* Madison: American History Research Center.
——— (1963) *American Doctors and German Universities.* Lincoln: University of Nebraska Press.
Braverman, H. (1974) *Labor and Monopoly Capital.* New York: Monthly Review Press.
Bremner, R. (1960) *American Philanthropy.* Chicago: University of Chicago Press.
Brody, D. (1969) *Steelworkers in America.* New York: Harper & Row.
Brown, E.R. (1979) *Rockefeller Medicine Men.* Los Angeles: University of California Press.
Bullock, H. (1967) *A History of Negro Education in the South.* Cambridge: Harvard University Press.
Carnegie, A. (1962) *The Gospel of Wealth and Other Essays.* Cambridge: Belknap Press of Harvard University.
Carnoy, M. (1974) *Education as Cultural Imperialism.* New York: David McKay.
Chapman, C. (1974) The Flexner Report. *Daedalus* 103: 105–17.
Chesney, A.M. (1963) *The Johns Hopkins Hospital and the Johns Hopkins University School of Medicine: A Chronicle:* vol. 3, *1905–1914.* Baltimore: Johns Hopkins University Press.
Cleaver, H. (1975) Origins of the Green Revolution. PhD Dissertation, Stanford University.
Codman, E.A (1913) The Product of a Hospital. *Surg. Gynec. Obstet.* 18: 491.
Corner, G. (1959) Johns Hopkins University and the Rockefeller Institute: Allies in the March of Science. *Occasional Papers by the Faculty and Friends of the Rockefeller Institute.* New York: Rockefeller Institute Press.
——— (1965) *A History of the Rockefeller Institute.* New York: Rockefeller Institute Press.
Cremin, L. (1964) *The Transformation of the School.* New York: Vintage Press.
Curti, M. (1963) *American Philanthropy Abroad: A History.* New Brunswick: Rutgers University Press.
Curti, M. and Nash, R. (1965) *Philanthropy in the Shaping of American Higher Education.* New Brunswick: Rutgers University Press.

Curti, M., Green, J., and Nash, R. (1963) Anatomy of Giving: Millionaires in the Late Nineteenth Century. *American Quarterly* 15: 416–35.

Cushing, H. (1949) *The Life of Sir William Osler.* New York: Oxford University Press.

De Kruif, P. (1962) *The Sweeping Wind: A Memoir.* New York: Harcourt, Brace & World.

Domhoff, G.W. (1970) *The Higher Circles.* New York: Vintage Books.

Duffus, R.L. and Holt, L.E., Jr. (1940) *L. Emmet Holt: Pioneer of a Children's Century.* New York: D. Appleton-Century.

Fleming, D. (1954) *William H. Welch and the Rise of American Medicine.* Boston: Little, Brown.

Flexner, A. (1908) *The American College: A Criticism.* New York: Century Publishing.

(1910) *Medical Education in the United States and Canada.* New York: Carnegie Foundation for the Advancement of Teaching.

(1912) *Medical Education in Europe.* New York: Carnegie Foundation for the Advancement of Teaching.

(1943) *Henry S. Pritchett: A Biography.* New York: Columbia University Press.

(1952) *Funds and Foundations.* New York: Harper & Bros.

(1959) Interview. Oral History Collection, Columbia University: New York.

(1960) *An Autobiography.* New York: Simon & Schuster.

Flexner, J. (1984) *An American Saga.* Boston: Little, Brown.

Flexner, S. (1929) *Addresses to Honor the Memory of Frederick T. Gates.* New York: Rockefeller Institute Press.

Flexner, S. and Flexner, J. (1966) *William H. Welch and the Heroic Age of American Medicine.* New York: Dover Publications.

Fosdick, R.B. (1952) *The Story of the Rockefeller Foundation.* New York: Harper & Bros.

(1956) *John D. Rockefeller, Jr.: A Portrait.* New York: Harper & Bros.

(1962) *Adventure in Giving.* New York: Harper & Bros.

Foucault, M. (1974) *The Birth of the Clinic.* New York: Pantheon.

Freidson, E. (1970) *Profession of Medicine.* New York: Dodd-Mead.

Freymann, J. (1974) *The American Health Care System: Its Genesis and Trajectory.* New York: Medcom Press.

References

Gates, F.T. (1911) *Notes on Homeopathy:* No. 3. New York: Rockefeller Foundation Archives.

(1916) *Addresses on the Tenth Anniversary of the Rockefeller Institute.* New York: Rockefeller Foundation Archives.

(1923) *Civilization and Disease.* New York: Rockefeller Foundation Archives.

(1927) *World Philanthropy.* New York: Rockefeller Foundation Archives.

(1977) *Chapters in My Life.* New York: Free Press.

General Education Board (1914) *The General Education Board: 1903–1914.* New York: General Education Board.

Goodspeed, T.W. (1916) *A History of the University of Chicago: The First Quarter Century.* Chicago: University of Chicago Press.

Harrell, G. (1973) Osler's Practice. *Bulletin of the History of Medicine* 47: 545–68.

Harrington, T. (1905) *The Harvard Medical School: A History, Narrative and Documentary, 1782–1905,* vol. 3. New York: Lewis Publishing.

Hirsch, E. (1966) *Frank Billings.* Chicago: University of Chicago Press.

Hofstadter, R and Hardy, D. (1952) *The Development and Scope of Higher Education in the United States.* New York: Columbia University Press.

Hofstadter, R. and Metzger, W. (1955) *The Development of Academic Freedom in the United States.* New York: Columbia University Press.

Hollis, E.V. (1939) *Philanthropic Foundations and Higher Education.* New York: Columbia University Press.

Holmes, B. (1906) The Hospital Problem. *Journal of the American Medical Association* 47: 318–20.

Horowitz, D. and Collier, P. (1975) *The Rockefellers: An American Dynasty.* New York: Holt, Rhinehart & Winston.

Hudson, R. (1972) Abraham Flexner in Perspective: American Medical Education 1865–1910. *Bulletin of the History of Medicine* 46: 545–61.

Jarcho, S. (1959) Medical Education in the United States: 1910–1956. *Journal of the Mt. Sinai Hospital* 26: 339–85.

Katz, M. (1968) *The Irony of Early School Reform.* Boston: Beacon

Press.

King, L. (1984) The Flexner Report of 1910. *Journal of the American Medical Association* 251:1079–086.

Kunitz, S. (1974) Professionalism and Social Control in the Progressive Era: The Case of the Flexner Report. *Social Problems* 22:16–27.

Lanksford, J. (1964) *Congress and the Foundations in the Twentieth Century.* River Falls: Wisconsin State University Press.

Latham, E. (ed.) (1949) *John D. Rockefeller: Robber Baron or Industrial Statesman?* Boston: D.C. Heath.

Leavell, U.W. (1930) *Philanthropy in Negro Education.* Nashville: George Peabody College for Teachers.

MacDonald, D. (1956) *The Ford Foundation: The Men and the Millions.* New York: Reynal & Co.

Marglin, S. (1974) What Do Bosses Do? *Review of Radical Political Economics* 6:33–60.

Markowitz, G. and Rosner, D. (1973) Doctors in Crisis. *American Quarterly* 25:83–107.

Morison, R.S. (1964) Foundations and Universities. *Daedalus* 93:1109–142.

Munger, D. (1968) Robert Brookings and the Flexner Report. *Journal of the History of Medicine.* 23:356–71.

Nevins, A. (1940) *John D. Rockefeller: The Heroic Age of American Enterprise,* vol. 2. New York: Charles Scribner.

——— (1953) *Study in Power: John D. Rockefeller, Industrialist and Philanthropist,* vol. 2. New York: Charles Scribner.

Parker, F. (1961) Abraham Flexner (1866–1959) and Medical Education. *Journal of Medical Education* 36:709–14.

Penfield, W. (1967) *The Difficult Art of Giving: The Epic of Allen Gregg.* Boston: Little, Brown.

Pollack, N. (1966) *The Populist Response to Industrial America.* New York: W.W. Norton.

Post, A. (1908) The Hospital in Relation to the Community. *Boston Medical and Surgical Journal* 158:823–28.

Prudden, T.M. (1927) *Biographical Sketches and Letters of T. Mitchell Prudden, M.D.* New Haven: Yale University Press.

Ratner, S. (ed.) (1953) *New Light on the History of the Great American Fortunes.* New York: Augustus Kelley.

References

Rayack, E. (1967) *Professional Power and American Medicine: The Economics of the AMA*. Cleveland: World Publishing.

Reverby, S. (1975) *Borrowing a Volume from Industry: A Study of Management Reform in American Hospitals, 1910–1945*. Draft.

Rockefeller, J.D. (1933) *Random Reminiscences of Men and Events*. New York: Doubleday, Doran.

Rockefeller, J.D., Jr. (1929) *Speeches to Honor the Memory of Frederick T. Gates*. New York: Rockefeller Institute Press.

Rothstein, W. (1972) *American Physicians in the 19th Century*. Baltimore: Johns Hopkins University Press.

Rudolph, F. (1962) *The American College and University*. New York: Vintage Press.

Sabin, F. (1934) *Franklin Paine Mall*. Baltimore: Johns Hopkins University Press.

Savage, H. (1953) *Fruit of an Impulse: 45 Years of the Carnegie Foundation, 1905–1950*. New York: Harcourt Brace.

Sears, J. (1922) *Philanthropy in the History of American Higher Education*. Washington, D.C.: United States Bureau of Education.

Shryock, R. (1936) *The Development of Modern Medicine*. Philadelphia: University of Pennsylvania Press.

——— (1953) *The Unique Influence of the Johns Hopkins University on American Medicine*. Copenhagen: Ejnar Munksgaard.

Smith, D. (1974) *Who Rules the Universities: An Essay in Class Analysis*. New York: Monthly Review Press.

Smith, W. (1974) The Development of American Medical Research and the Influence of John D. Rockefeller. *Journal of the Oklahoma State Medical Association* 67:146–55.

Spring, J. (1973) *Education and the Rise of the Corporate State*. Boston: Beacon Press.

Starr, Paul (1983) *The Social Transformation of American Medicine*. New York: Basic Books.

Stevens, R. (1972) *American Medicine and the Public Interest*. New Haven: Yale University Press.

Stone, K. (1974) The Origin of Job Structures in the Steel Industry. *Review of Radical Political Economics* 6:61–97.

Storr, R. (1966) *Harper's University: The Beginnings*. Chicago: University of Chicago Press.

Sullivan, M. (1930) *Our Times: The United States 1900–1925*, vol 3.

New York: Charles Scribner.

Tarbell, I. (1904) *History of the Standard Oil Company*. New York: Macmillan.

Tucker, W.J. (1891) The Gospel of Wealth. *Andover Review* 15: 631-45.

Turshen, M. (1975) The Political Economy of Health with a Case Study of Tanzania. PhD Dissertation, University of Sussex.

United States Bureau of the Census (1960) *Historical Statistics of the United States: Colonial Times to 1957.* Washington D.C.: U.S. Government Printing Office.

Veysey, L. (1965) *The Emergence of the American University*. Chicago: University of Chicago Press.

Wall, J. (1970) *Andrew Carnegie*. New York: Oxford University Press.

Wasserman, H. (1972) *Harvey Wasserman's History of the United States.* New York: Harper & Row.

Weaver, W. (1967) *United States Philanthropic Foundations.* New York: Harper & Row.

Weinstein, J. (1968) *The Corporate Ideal in the Liberal State.* Boston: Beacon Press.

Winslow, C.E.A. (1929) *The Life of Hermann Biggs.* Philadelphia: Lea & Febiger.

Index

affiliations between medical schools and universities 38
Agassiz, Louis 21
Aldrich, Nelson 129
allopathy 38, 39–40
American Association for Labor Legislation 138
American Baptist Education Society 27, 37, 77
American Bar Association 106
American Linseed Oil Co. 77
American Medical Association 66, 68–9, 98–100, 105–06, 108, 111, 112, 120, 122, 138, 150, 161, 164–65
American Ship Building Corp. 77
Anderson, Martin B. 26
Andrews, E. Benjamin 30
anti-contagionism 80
Armstrong, Samuel 8
Association of American Physicians 66
Astor, John J. 138
Atlantic, The 118

Baker, George 22
Baldwin, William 9
Barker, Llewellys F. 141, 159–60
Bellevue Hospital 93, 94
Bellevue Medical College 65
Bevan, Arthur Dean 38, 110–11, 164
Biggs, Herman 65, 67
Billings, John Shaw 118
Billroth, Theodore 106
Breslau University 142
Brookings, Robert 162
Brown University 19, 23, 30, 103
Bryan, William Jennings 78
Bulletin Number Four 1, 97, 111, 122, 124, 127, 150, 171; *see also* Flexner Report
Butler, Nicholas Murray 74
Buttrick, Wallace 29, 132, 165, 170

Cahoon, Emma Lucille 26
capital and labor 77
Carnegie, Andrew 5, 11, 13–18, 23, 29, 32–3, 74, 92–3, 97, 106, 110, 118, 121, 126, 132

Carnegie Foundation for the Advancement of Teaching 1, 4, 6, 25, 35, 93, 97-8, 99-100, 103-04, 107, 111, 112, 118, 119-20, 123, 125, 126, 131, 132, 138, 143, 147, 162, 164, 165, 170
Carnegie Institution 74
Carnegie Laboratory 93
Carnegie Steel Corporation 11
'Carnegie Unit' 98
Carrell, Alexis 89
cerebro-spinal meningitis 89-90
Chicago 37, 119
Chicago Tribune 119
Chicago University 5, 23, 27, 36-52, 53, 75, 96, 130, 141, 162, 165
Civil War 134
clinicians 147, 149-50, 151-54, 155-59
Codman, E.A. 137
Cole, Rufus 90
College of Physicians and Surgeons 54
Colorado Fuel and Iron 77
Columbia-Presbyterian Medical Center 166
Columbia University 23, 54, 60, 72, 96, 125, 130, 162, 164, 166
Colwell, N.P. 108
Commission on Industrial Relations 132
Congress of the United States 129-30
contagionism 80
Cornell, Ezra 15
Cornell University 22, 97, 162
Council on Medical Education 99-100, 105-06, 107-08, 110, 111, 119, 122, 161, 164
Councilman, William T. 104, 105
Coxey's Army 11
Curie, Marie 93
Curry, J.L.M. 11
Cushing, Harvey 154

Davis Coke and Coal Co. 77
De Kruif, Paul 86-8, 90
Dennis, Frederick 92
diptheria antitoxin 65
disease, theories on 78-84

Eastman, George 22, 23
education: higher 19-25; medical *see* medical education; scientific 21-3
El Paso News 119
elective system 20
Eliot, Charles 20, 21, 89, 90, 102-03, 105, 163
Europe, medical systems in 166-69

Fifth Avenue Baptist Church of Minneapolis 26
Fifth Avenue Baptist Church of New York 64
Flexner, Abraham 1, 5, 6, 36, 37, 101-17, 118, 119-20, 121, 123-27, 132, 139, 140, 141, 145-46, 147-51, 152, 162, 164, 165, 171-72, 173-74
Flexner, Simon 54, 67, 75, 87, 88, 89-90, 95, 97, 102, 103, 107, 121, 125, 140, 142, 143, 147
Flexner Report 1, 3-4, 5, 6, 35, 97, 110-17, 118-27, 128, 131, 139, 140-41, 142, 146, 150, 162; *see also* Bulletin Number Four
Flexner Report of 1911 *see* 1911 Report
Foucault, Michel 137

Index

foundations 7–10, 13–16, 18, 25, 128–33
Franklin, Benjamin 7
full-time plan 139–44, 141–61, 162–66, 167, 168, 171, 173

Gary, Elbert H. 138
Gates, Frederick T. 5, 6, 12, 26–34, 37, 39, 40–1, 43–5, 47–9, 50–2, 53–9, 70, 72, 75, 76–9, 82–8, 89–90, 94, 95, 106–07, 109, 124–26, 139, 141–42, 143–46, 147, 150, 154–59, 163, 166, 167–71, 172–74
General Education Board 4, 5, 6, 25, 28–34, 35, 109, 124, 126, 129, 131–32, 138, 139, 142, 145, 148, 159, 160, 162–66, 168, 169–75
geographic full-time system 139, 163
germ theory of disease 79–84
Gilman, Daniel Coit 21, 101, 103
Goodspeed, Thomas W. 40, 41–2, 43, 44, 45–7, 51, 56, 57
'Gospel of Wealth' 13–18, 92
Gould, Jay 23
Granges and Farmers Associations 11
Gross National Product (GNP) 11

Hale, Edward Everett 134
Halstead, William 134, 156
Hampton Institute 8
Hanna, Marc 23
Harper, William Rainey 23, 38–9, 40, 41–2, 43, 45–7, 48–50, 54, 55, 141
Harvard Medical School 63, 72, 94, 119, 162, 163, 173
Harvard University 20, 21, 22, 60, 75, 102–03, 130
Haymarket Massacre 11
health insurance 138
Hearst Press 89
Hektoen, Ludwig 38
Herter, Christian A. 65–6, 67
Holt, L. Emmett 64–5, 67, 70, 93, 95
homeopathy 39
Homestead Strike 11
Hopkins, Johns 15, 101, 133
Hospital of the Rockefeller Institute 134, 151
hospitals 133–38
Huntington, Elon O. 54–5
Hurd, Henry M. 154
Huxley, Thomas H. 58

Industrial Workers of the World 11
industrialization 10–11
Ingals, E. Fletcher 38–9, 42, 46, 49
Institute for Advanced Study 174
International Harvester 69
Iowa University 162, 172–74
Iveagh, Lord 62

Janeway, Theodore 160
Jenner Institute of Preventive Medicine 62
Jessup, Morris K. 30
Jobling, James W. 87
Jochmann, Georg 87
Johns Hopkins Hospital 94, 125, 134, 143, 144, 148
Johns Hopkins Medical School 55, 93–4, 95, 102, 106, 118, 119, 124, 125, 126, 139, 141, 142, 143–48, 154–55, 158–60, 162–65, 173

187

Johns Hopkins University 21, 101, 130, 159, 160, 165
Journal of the American Medical Association 68, 120–21, 161

Kelly, Howard 134, 154, 156
Kenyon College 23
Kirkland, James H. 99–100
Klebs, Edwin 38
Knoxville (Tennessee) Sentinel 119
Koch, Robert 87, 93
Koch Institute 57
Kruse, Walther 87

labor activity 11
laboratory scientists 140–41, 142, 147, 150, 152
Lafayette College 22
Lake Forest College 38
Landis Decision 88, 130
Lawrence, Abbott 21
Lawrence School 21
Lehigh University 22
Library of Congress 105, 108
Lincoln School 174
Los Angeles Daily Times 119
Low, Seth 60–4, 71
Ludlow Massacre 88–9, 132–33, 171
Ludwig, Carl 141

McCall's 130
McCormick, Harold R. 64, 69–70
McCormick Institute for the Study of Infectious Diseases 70, 74
MacDonald, Sir William 94
McGill Medical School 94–7, 128, 162
McGill University 107
Mall, Franklin P. 106, 141

Mann, Horace 19
Marglin, Stephen 136
Maryland Medical Journal 68
Massachusetts Institute of Technology (MIT) 22, 23, 97
Mather, Cotton 7
medical education 103–17, 118–27, 128, 137, 139–61, 162–69, 171–75
Medical Notes and Queries 123
Medical Practice Act 1858 133
Medical Record 68, 121
Medical Society of the State of New York 122
'Medical Trust' 111
medicine, state of 2–3, 54, 56–7, 79–84
medicine as religion 84–5
Milbank Foundation 138
Modern Hospital 136
Morgan, J.P. 72, 132, 138
Munsterberg, Hugo 105
Murphy, Starr J. 44, 57, 59–60, 65, 72–3, 76, 143, 145

Nashville University 8
National Association of Manufacturers 138
National Education Association 131–32
Nature 119–20
Nevins, Allan 91
New York City Board of Health 66
New York Evening Journal 89
New York Evening Post 67
New York Medical Journal 68
New York State Journal of Medicine 121–23
New York Times 67–8, 119
New York University 23
1911 Report 148–54

Index

Nobel Prize 89-90, 91
North American Review 14
Novy, Frederick 86
Nuttall, George 60-1, 62, 63

Ogden, Robert C. 8
Omaha Bee 119
Osler, William 45, 53, 54-7, 78, 83, 87, 88, 94-5, 97, 134, 150-54, 155, 156-57
osteopathy 45
Oxford University 150

Pall Mall Gazette 14
Pasteur, Louis 56, 57, 87, 90
Pasteur Institute 57, 60, 61, 83, 93
pay wards 149
Peabody, George F. 7-8, 30, 170
Peabody Fund 7-8, 9, 30, 34
Peabody Normal College 8
Pennsylvania University 22
Perkins, Lucia Fowler 26
philanthropy 7-8, 12-18; retail v. wholesale 27-8; *see also* foundations
Phipps Institute for the Study of Tuberculosis 74
Pillsbury, George 27
pneumonia 87, 90
political status quo 82-3, 121-23, 135-38
Poor Laws 133
population 10
Populism 78
Pritchett, Henry 5, 97-8, 103-06, 107, 118, 121, 123-26, 162, 165-66
Prudden, T. Mitchell 60, 62, 63, 64, 65, 67, 71, 93
Pullman Strike 11

Randall, Blanchard 143

Remsen, Ira 103, 150
Rennssalear Polytechnical Institute 21, 23
Review of Reviews 18
Rice, Allen Thorndike 14
Rochester Theological Seminary 26
Rochester University 23, 26, 162
Rockefeller, John D. Jr 28, 53, 59-60, 64-5, 66-7, 69-74, 76, 86, 91, 93, 105, 129, 132, 145, 158, 171, 174
Rockefeller, John D. Sr 5, 11, 12, 13, 18, 23, 27-8, 29, 31-2, 37, 39, 40-1, 43-5, 47, 49, 50, 51, 57, 58-9, 68, 69, 71-5, 78, 87-9, 91, 92, 94, 125, 126, 130, 132, 138, 142, 143, 158, 170
Rockefeller Foundation 129-30, 132, 167-68
Rockefeller General Education Board *see* General Education Board
Rockefeller Institute for Medical Research 5-6, 35, 50, 53-75, 76, 85-91, 93, 95-7, 102, 103, 107, 121, 124-25, 131, 134, 142, 143, 146-7, 175
Rockefeller Sanitary Commission 35, 130
Rockefeller University 53
Royal College of Physicians and Surgeons 62
Rush Medical College 5, 36-52, 53, 58, 75
Russell Sage Foundation 138
Ryerson, Martin 46, 49

Sage, Mrs Russell 23
Sears, Barnas 7, 8
Senn, Nicholas 38

Shaw, Albert 18
Sheffield, Joseph 21
Sheffield Scientific School 21, 101
Simmons, George H. 106
Slater, John F. 8–9
Slater Fund 8–9
Small, Albion 24
Smith, Theobald 65, 66, 67, 75
Smithson, James 7
Smithsonian Institution 7
Social Medicine 80–1, 82
Southern Education Board 28, 29
Standard Oil Company 12, 27, 32, 59, 88–9, 130, 132–33
Stanford, Leland 15
Stevens Institute of Technology 23
Storr, Richard 38

Tarbell, Ida 88, 130
Thayer, William S. 160
Tribune 67
Tucker, Henry St George 9
Tucker, William Jewett 16–18
Tuskeegee Institute 8

United States Steel 11
University Record 48

urbanization 10

Vanderbilt University 99–100, 162
Vassar College 102
Virchow, Rudolf 80
Von Pirquet, Clemens 142–43, 148

Walsh, Frank 132
Wannamaker, John 8
Ward, Lester 24
Washington, Booker T. 8
Washington and Lee University 9
Washington University 162, 163
Wayland, Francis 19
wealth 11–12; *see also* 'Gospel of Wealth'
Welch, William H. 60–7, 69, 71, 72–3, 75, 88, 89, 92–3, 95–7, 102, 103, 106–07, 124–25, 140, 142–48, 154–56, 157, 159
West Point 21
Western Maryland Railroad 77
Western Reserve University 96
Workman's Compensation 138
World War I 167, 168, 172

Yale University 21, 22, 130, 162